# Asian American Identities, Relationships, and Post-Migration Legacies

W0091299

Bringing together the personal and professional narratives of Asian American family therapists, this book offers insight into the Asian American experience through systemic theory and frameworks, individual and community stories, and clinical considerations.

The Asian American experience is still a largely invisible and unknown one, especially in the field of marriage and family therapy. With a contextual lens, this book highlights how understanding family migration legacies and individual generational status relative to time, place, and context is critical to doing meaningful work with Asian Americans. Filled with thought-provoking case studies and reflective questions, chapters discuss the impact of stereotyping on mental health; the historical and present ways that Asian American racialization invisibilizes individual and collective experiences; shame associated with bicultural identity, gender, generational trauma, media representations; and more. Each chapter bridges these ideas to clinical practice while concurrently centering the voices and experiences of Asian American therapists.

This book is essential reading for marriage and family therapists and other mental health clinicians who want to deepen their understanding of, relationship with, and clinical support for the Asian Americans in their lives, whether friends, colleagues, supervisees, or clients.

**Jessica ChenFeng, PhD, LMFT** (she/her), daughter of immigrants from Taiwan, is a systemic therapist, consulting with academic, healthcare, and church organizations to improve the well-being of people within their communities. Her work centers around social contextual intersections of race, gender, generation, trauma, and spirituality. She is an associate professor of marriage and family therapy at Fuller Theological Seminary.

**Lana Kim, PhD, LMFT** (she/her), daughter of immigrants from South Korea, is a systemic therapist, supervisor, and educator with a background in medical family therapy. Her clinical and research focus includes contextual issues in teaching and supervision, relational parenting, sociocultural and socio-emotional attunement in couple therapy, and collaborative care practices. She is an associate professor and the program director for the Marriage, Couple, and Family Therapy program at Lewis & Clark College in Portland, Oregon.

Editors/authors ChenFeng and Kim have created a gem. It is not a how-to manual. Instead, it is an invitation to reflect upon Asian and Asian American identities, (in)visibility, race, and the contextualization of a highly minoritized and stereotyped people. Authors draw from their own varied experiences as Asian Americans, immigrants, multi-ethnic folks, and marriage and family therapists, while harnessing critical tools of scholarly inquiry. This book meets an urgent need for practitioners and readers to understand historical and recent trauma, shame, resilience while equipping themselves to understand, support, intervene and advocate. I recommend this book most highly to all systemic therapists and trainees.

**Mudita Rastogi, PhD, LMFT**, Clinical Professor and
McCormick Tribune Foundation Chair in
Family Therapy, MSMFT Program, The Family
Institute at Northwestern University

This book is a necessary read for any mental health professional. The book educates us about the cultural identity of Asian Americans within a historical, sociopolitical context while delving into the personal stories of marriage and family therapists and providing clinical guidance for working with Asian Americans. More than being an educational text for those unfamiliar with Asian American history, this book seems like home and a safe place for Asian Americans. The authors truly SEE you, all of you.

**DeAnna Harris-McKoy, PhD, LMFT**,
Associate Professor/ SMFT Program Director at
Northern Illinois University

The voices of Asian American therapists provide a rich, nuanced view into the lives of diverse Asian American clients. Visibilizing the diversity of Asian American couples and families benefits all therapists that serve couples and families, regardless of ethnic origins. Learning how diverse values, beliefs, and practices are evidenced across different families can help all providers develop hypotheses about cultural and contextual factors that might be exerting influences on those whom they serve. The ability to witness factors specific to Asian American families is a two-fold gift that the authors in this volume provide: Asian American readers will experience representation and validation; non-Asian American readers will have access and deepen awareness of a host of lived experiences that might otherwise be inaccessible to them. The focus on clinical concepts and skills will be profoundly helpful to those serving Asian American clients.

**Melanie Domenech-Rodriguez, Ph.D., ABPP**,
Professor, Utah State University and
Editor, Family Process

# Asian American Identities, Relationships, and Post-Migration Legacies

Reflections from Marriage and Family Therapists

Edited by Jessica ChenFeng and Lana Kim

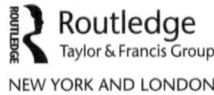

Routledge
Taylor & Francis Group

NEW YORK AND LONDON

<< Designed cover image: Sole
30"x40" / 76x101cm
Hyunah Kim
www.hyunahkim.com
Drenched in the optimism of yellow and the tranquility of light purple, 'Sole' stands as an embodiment of hope, ambition, and pride. This abstract modern painting delves into minimal expressionism to create a captivating narrative. The radiant yellow whispers of dreams and aspirations, while the calming light purple exudes a sense of pride, rooted in quiet confidence. This interaction of hues crafts a symbolic dialogue, reflecting the human journey from dreaming to achieving. The simplicity of its design makes 'Sole' an engaging and inspiring addition to any contemporary art collection.

First published 2025
by Routledge
605 Third Avenue, New York, NY 10158

and by Routledge
4 Park Square, Milton Park, Abingdon, Oxon, OX14 4RN

*Routledge is an imprint of the Taylor & Francis Group, an informa business*

© 2025 selection and editorial matter, Jessica ChenFeng and Lana Kim; individual chapters, the contributors

The right of Jessica ChenFeng and Lana Kim to be identified as the authors of the editorial material, and of the authors for their individual chapters, has been asserted in accordance with sections 77 and 78 of the Copyright, Designs and Patents Act 1988.

ISBN: 978-1-032-34339-6 (hbk)
ISBN: 978-1-032-34338-9 (pbk)
ISBN: 978-1-003-32159-0 (ebk)

DOI: 10.4324/9781003321590

Typeset in Times New Roman
by Deanta Global Publishing Services, Chennai, India

前人種樹後人乘涼.

One generation plants the trees, in whose shade another generation rests.
*Chinese proverb*

Through my parents' enduring love and steadfast hope,
Because of my husband's partnership and mutual support,
And for our children and their children.
JCF

My parents for their unwavering love and endless sacrifice
My husband for walking with me
My children for their world, today and tomorrow
LK

# Contents

# Introduction

*Jessica ChenFeng and Lana Kim*

As Asian North American co-authors and co-editors, this book is as much for you, our reader and for our Asian American clinician colleagues, as much as it is for us. In our years of teaching and supervising in the field of marital and family therapy, it seems that the beckoning of most into the field is deeply personal. This seems especially so for therapists of color and is certainly true for us. We witness mental health needs in our own racial and ethnic communities, we have personal experiences of relational rupture in our own family systems, and we are pained by the invisibility and minoritization of our racial groups within our professional fields. Who we are shapes what we do and why we do it. That is what this book is about.

Through dreaming up the vision for this book and these months of writing, we have carried closely with us the Asian American students, clients, and colleagues who have left their imprint on our personal and professional lives. We have seen reflected in ourselves your stories of resilience in the face of being unseen and neglected. We continue to persist with you to engage in the challenging work of staying present to the layers of discomfort and growth required to hear our collective voice. Together as a community, we hold dear our own identities, relationships, and post-migration legacies that have shaped who we are today.

## Timeliness in Context

According to the Pew Research Center (Budiman & Ruiz, 2021), single race, non-Hispanic Asians are currently the fastest-growing racial and ethnic group in the U.S., and overall, they make up 7% of the country's population. As early as the 16th century, Filipino, Chinese, and South Asian sailors and indentured servants came to the Americas by way of the Spanish galleons (Aráullo, 2023; Okihiro, 2015). Formal records of Asian immigration date back to the 19th century, with Japanese Americans who arrived to work on plantations and Chinese Americans who helped build the transcontinental railroad. But the largest documented period of migration was during the post-1965 immigration reform that

DOI: 10.4324/9781003321590-1

lifted quotas and head taxes on the numbers of people who were permitted to migrate to the U.S. from Asian countries. Since that time, the Asian American population in the U.S. has continued to increase among refugees, immigrants seeking greater social and economic opportunities, and U.S.-born children.

Asian Americans are a highly diverse group with over 20 ethnicities represented in Census surveys (Budiman & Ruiz, 2021). Despite this, in the broader American societal context, the diversity among Asian Americans has often been overlooked, and their realities have been invisibilized or discussed in monolithic and stereotypic ways. This pattern of marginalization has also been observed within the marriage and family therapy (MFT) field. It is only more recently that in the aftermath of rising anti-Asian hate and the post-2020 racial justice movement, as well as the rising global trend of Asian media, pop music, and food, that interest and regard for the realities of Asian American lives is increasing.

Representation and how any group is represented matters when it comes to influencing societal beliefs about who belongs and is valued in society. It matters because these shape our perceptions about whose lives have worth and significance. Ideas about Asian Americans have been largely narrated through a racialized lens rooted in systemic racism. This has left Asian Americans outside of U.S. consciousness unless it is to associate them with mass level political events such as the attack on Pearl Harbor and the COVID-19 pandemic that directly stoke the underlying, long-standing, Western anxieties of Asians as threat—an ideology that is rooted in the 19th-century yellow peril metaphor (Hsu, 2015). Media representations similarly cast Asian Americans under this lens of otherized threat or as foreign bodies. These processes intentionally maintain a skewed picture of who Asian Americans are, and this has shaped our marginalization in society.

In social discourse, Asian Americans continue to get highlighted for their visible phenotypic differences and are either considered as forever foreigners or objectified as a model minority. Both of these dehumanize with one stereotype suggesting Asian Americans are not full members of U.S. society while the other suggests Asians are only accepted and valued in American society if they are able to fulfill white society's standards for minoritized groups. What gets left out are the histories, struggles, perspectives, strengths, and identities that Asian Americans hold as individuals as well as the relational legacies that exist within our families.

Along with the growing U.S. Asian American population, we imagine that there will only continue to be increasing numbers of Asian Americans who engage with the MFT field, both as future clinicians and clients. At the time of writing and editing this book, we are honored that it would be the first in the field of marriage and family therapy to center the experiences of Asian Americans— both client and therapist—and to offer clinical reflections that are contextually and systemically situated. We hope for this book to punctuate the curiosity about Asian American lives with a critically conscious understanding of some of the most intimate and meaningful parts of our lives: our relationships with ourselves, our families, and our cultural and racial selves.

A book of this kind is only possible because of the work that was already done by Asian American elders of the MFT field and our Asian American colleagues in other disciplines, including clinical psychology and social work. We also recognize our Black, Indigenous, and Latinx MFT colleagues whose powerful voices through decades of leadership, service, and transformative scholarship have shaped our field. Your courage, sacrifice, and humility have paved the way for us to keep hoping for and working toward a more equitable and inclusive mutual reality for ourselves, our trainees, and clients.

## Purpose and Function of Book

Because the literature on Asian American families predominantly focuses on Asians as first-generation, immigrant families, the majority of family science research has been done around acculturation and assimilation processes, hierarchical parent-child relationships, and generational conflicts. Furthermore, the macrosystemic factors influencing these microsystemic processes have been minimally discussed. It is false to assume that today's Asian American families are only first and second generation. There are many families who have lived in the U.S. since the 19th century whose stories have not been shared, and a large number of children of first-generation immigrants are now parenting the third generation. Not surprisingly, the context surrounding their experiences differs significantly from the first generation of post-1965 immigrants. There is a need for more literature for and about families across the Asian American diaspora in the U.S. that feature their varied experiences, histories, and realities in today's contemporary context.

There is also a long-standing bias to equate Asian Americans with East Asian Americans, historically leaving out South and Southeast Asian Americans (Nadal, 2019). This exclusionary bias perpetuates discrimination and prejudice, and it needs to be challenged. Our desire is for all Asian American readers to feel acknowledged and invited to participate in the dialogue that will unfold across the pages to follow. Thus, in this book, Asian Americans include South, Southeast, and East Asian American identities. It is our hope that this book contributes to expanding the ways that we talk, view, and understand Asian American lives within the field of marriage and family therapy.

We also want to bring attention to the title of the book, that this is about Asian American identities, relationships, and *post-migration legacies*. Asian American lives lived in the U.S. are shaped not only by the actual experiences of migration but by all that was left behind and the new life—whether chosen or forced—that begins on Turtle Island (North America). After migration, the histories of settler colonialism, legacies of white cisheteropatriarchy, and Asian American racialization are thrust into the shaping of the Asian American self and family.

The book is unique in several ways. It is written by a collection of Asian American marriage and family therapy scholars and practitioners about diverse Asian American family issues and relational processes that relate to family therapy. This book offers a place where relational values and ethics common to Asian ethnicities are appreciated rather than pathologized for the contrast it presents to dominant, white American culture. Each chapter addresses particular theoretical, social, and historical contexts that affect the Asian American experience and also discusses the influence of family migration legacies. While each chapter may refer to similar concepts that are common to the broad Asian American experience, this book is different from a standard academic text in that it is written in a memoir style that invites the authors to bring in their own personal identities and honors their insights and perspectives to humanize our discussion about the variations of Asian American experience. As you read through this text, we invite you to sit with us and feel seen and known (especially our Asian American readers) as you seek to see, feel, and know who we are, and not just know about us.

## Intended Audience and Recommended Use

For a long time, our field has needed a book like this, and we wonder if now is the time for it to come together in the way that it has. This book is actualized because of the nurturing of relationships among Asian American MFT friends, mentors/mentees, and colleagues over time. We met each other as academics at conferences, invited one another to speak for our classes or institutions, got to know each other's research, served on dissertation committees, and have written together over the years. We dream of you, our readers, as being able to foster and deepen your relationships through dialogue about this book; may it facilitate conversations of shared humility, compassion, and curiosity that ignite your own visions for intergenerational healing and hope.

I wonder about how a book like this could have shaped my own experience (Jessica) through years of graduate school training. I can remember one of the few articles on Asian American issues that was assigned during my doctoral studies. To this day, even if my own ethnic identity was not reflected in this article, I remember the impact Pyke's (2000) article "The Normal American Family as an Interpretive Structure of Family Life among Grown Children of Korean and Vietnamese Immigrants" had on my personal, relational, and racialized self. We read this article in a doctoral course where I was one of the few Asian American students in class. I recall feeling both a vulnerability and a sense of being more visible and known. I wondered what my mostly white peers thought about Asian Americans and what this meant about their thoughts about me. I was so used to my and our experience being unknown that this peering into the inner world of Asian American identity left me feeling exposed. I also worried and wondered: Did they know the difference between Korean, Vietnamese, and my own Taiwanese identity? Did they know that this research article was not a comprehensive discussion of all Asian American experience? I felt the burden of having to clarify, correct, and represent Asian Americanness rightly somehow.

Similar to Jessica, having a published text like this that seeks to legitimize and make known the lived realities and experiences of Asian Americans would have been formative to my (Lana) graduate training. I believe it would have also helped me feel affirmed in my belonging as an emerging professional in the field. It was more uncommon than not to have assigned readings like Pyke's (2000) article and adjacent discussions that explicitly included Asian American realities. Therefore, when classroom and training experiences centered on Asian American experiences, I remember bracing for the vulnerability about what might get portrayed, how tokenized I might feel, and vacillating between whether or not to defend, explain, and translate the constructed narrative. I had no reason to trust that what the class would read and how they would interpret it would be validating and humanizing because of how narrow the collection of stories typically were about Asian Americans. Much of my professional socialization was seeing Asian Americans and what affected them be invisibilized, ignored, or misunderstood, and this contributed to me struggling to figure out where and how Asian Americans at large fit into the field of family therapy and larger context of mental health.

Books like this promote community and membership for the growing numbers of Asian American professionals in the field. The book is written for Asian American family therapists, educators, students, and those who are interested in being a part of *re-membering* how Asian American families, individuals, and their experiences are represented in society. In envisioning this book, we have thought fondly of and empathically for our Asian American colleagues, and past and present students in the field who know the feeling of being one of the few or only. We hope that this book reduces the burden of having to personally represent and make our stories known. We long for us to feel less alone and more interconnected. Whether or not we ever get the chance to meet, we know that there are Asian American therapists sharing in this collective hope and burden of Asian American joy and liberation.

We are grateful for our non-Asian American readers and your investment in Asian American identity and the intersections with your unique cultural and racial identities. We hope and trust that your open engagement with this book will lead to more meaningful and mutual connections with your Asian American friends, family, colleagues, students, and clients.

This book is not a "how to" guide for working with Asian American persons and families in therapy. Because it centers Asian Americans as the reader, it assumes that there are some cultural concepts that will be viscerally resonant with the Asian American experience broadly, and thus we intentionally do not explain Asian values and processes that may be familiar to persons who identify within Asian ethnicities. While we acknowledge that the experiences and concepts the authors discuss are not exhaustive and may not be representative of all Asian Americans living in the U.S., our hope is that readers will be able to take the concepts and apply them to the specific ways in which they present in their own and their clients' lives.

In addition to being written for clinicians and serving as a resource for creating community around the Asian American identity and experience, this text is also recommended for inclusion in family therapy, professional mental health counseling, social work, and psychology courses related to equity and diversity, family systems, lifespan development, couple relationships, parent-child relationships, and practical applications. It can also be used in group practice or consultation contexts to allow for clinicians to engage in dialogue with one another.

Something important we would like to remind readers is that in a book such as this, we understand that the discussion of Asian American experience can include potentially activating issues. Our families and communities live with past and on-going personal, societal, and racialized trauma. We hope and trust that you will seek communities of support, places to process, debrief, and connect, and the discernment to pause and pace yourself.

## A Third-Order Lens

First- and second-order thinking are familiar concepts to systems therapists. Even if each chapter of this book may not directly reference a third-order lens, the overarching hope is that the content of this book propels us to assuming a third-order posture. We believe that third-order thinking, introduced by Theresa McDowell, characterizes a critically important shift in the field that "requires us to attune to sociocultural experience and adopt perspectives that include frameworks for understanding societal context and power" (McDowell, Knudson-Martin, Bermudez, 2019, p. 12). While attending to and valuing the frames that first- and second-order thinking give us, we see these lenses as embedded within larger systems—that each unique Asian American family system and dynamic functions inside of and breathes the air of a larger U.S. dominant racialized system (systems within systems)—this is third-order thinking. As therapists taking on a third-order perspective, we pay close attention to how these larger systems (historical, social, political, etc.) organize what we notice, what clients respond to and why they react, and how we understand families. We invite you to consider how this book supports the development of a third-order perspective.

## The Authors and the Chapters

We hope you will listen closely to each and all narratives in this book and the nuanced complexities of Asian ethnicities and generations represented in our authors' lived experiences. We are grateful to our colleagues who have trusted us with the vision of this book to share their personal and professional selves with the community.

The book has nine chapters, segmented into three parts. Part I, *Contextualizing Silence and Invisibility*, discusses historical and contextual constraints and reasons about how and why Asian Americans have experienced silencing and invisibility. In Chapter 1, Saliha Bava unpacks the racialization of Asian American invisibilization with a transcontextual lens. In Chapter 2, Hoa Nguyen dives into the construction of common Asian American stereotypes of the model minority, honorary whiteness, and forever foreigner. Chapter 3 (Jessica and Lana) gives voice to racialized gender and the grief around how Asian American femininity/masculinity is constructed.

Part II, *Resistance, Resilience, and Imagined Possibilities*, highlights the ways Asian Americans have pushed back against the silence and invisibility and are imagining and expanding pathways to living beyond limiting narratives. In Chapter 4, Michael Chen situates Asian American bodies in context and envisions re-humanizing stories. Chapter 5 (Lana and Jessica) explores cross-generational racism and the critical use of a socioculturally attuned clinical lens to amplify resilient possibilities. In Chapter 6, Ulash Thakore-Dunlap and Bowbay Feng reframe therapy as activism and how therapists can cultivate healing spaces.

In light of the post-migration legacies passed on to us, the last part, Part III, *Transforming our Inheritance*, takes readers through clinically nuanced conversations that re-imagine a future for Asian American identities and relationships. In Chapter 7, Natalie Hsieh shares her grounded theory research recasting shame as a valuable witness to Asian American relational pain, disconnection, and attachment needs and proposes a model for shame resilience. Wonyoung Cho, in Chapter 8, beautifully invites us to consider how relational ethics are at the heart of the Asian American intergenerational family system. The book concludes with Chapter 9, where Amy Tuttle brings a multi-generational reflection on the enduring impact of family migration legacies.

Finally, we introduce you to these dear colleagues and friends, whose collective voice of academic, clinical, and personal reflections brings the vision of this book to life. In order of chapter authorship:

**Saliha Bava, PhD, LMFT** (she/they), born and raised in Delhi, India, arrived at Virginia Tech, Blacksburg, VA, in the mid-1990s for her doctoral studies. Currently residing in New York City, she consults with couples, companies, and communities, including Asians and Asian American clients and professionals. She is the first Indian to receive the *AFTA Distinguished Contribution to Family Therapy Theory and Practice Award* (2023). As a professor of marriage and family therapy at Mercy University, Taos Institute board member and associate, and a co-founding board member of the International Certificate in Collaborative-Dialogic Practices, she conducts international trainings, including in Asia. She focuses on expanding relational intelligence for an inclusive world by harnessing the power of play and dialogue. Performative methodologies, relational play, hyperlinked thinking, and dialogue guide her academic and social activism, which aims to unsettle dominant discourses regarding research, social justice, and identity. She co-authored *The Relational Workplace* and *The Relational Book for Parenting* with her partner Mark Greene and is a co-editor of the forthcoming *Routledge International Handbook of Postmodern Therapies*. She expresses her intersectional identities through playful interactions with her partner and son and experimental fusion cooking. Learn more at SalihaBava.com Email: drbava@gmail.com. Follow IG @drbava_nyc

**Hoa N. Nguyen, PhD, LMFT** (she/her), was born in Saigon, Vietnam, and raised in the Atlanta area of Georgia. At a young age, she immigrated with her family as part of a Vietnamese refugee resettlement program. Her clinical work and research has been with queer Asian Americans and exploring the in-between spaces of being not quite American and not quite Asian. Her research interests focus on the intersection of cultural and sexual identity and cultural humility in family therapy training and education. Her pedagogy centers on helping graduate family therapy students learn how to facilitate and engage in transformative dialogue. Currently, she teaches courses on social constructionism, ethics, and diversity, inclusion, and social justice in family therapy. She is an associate professor of marriage and family therapy at Valdosta State University and resides in Georgia with her partner and their cat and corgi pup. She enjoys crocheting, karaoke, and spending time with her nieces and nephews.

**Jessica ChenFeng, PhD, LMFT** (she/her), was born and raised in the San Gabriel Valley of Southern California. She is the daughter of immigrants from Southern Taiwan, who arrived in SoCal by way of Buenos Aires, Manhattan, Ann Arbor, and Seattle. She has been practicing for almost 20 years and her clinical work with Asian Americans has largely been with second-generation populations and with Asian/Asian American physicians. She has also mentored Asian American MFT students across academic institutions and minority-serving organizations. Additionally, she consults with academic, healthcare, and church organizations to improve the well-being of people within their communities. Her research and clinical work center around social contextual intersections of race, gender, generation, trauma, and spirituality. She is an associate professor of marriage and family therapy at Fuller Theological Seminary and has never stopped living in Southern California, where she resides with her spouse and two children. Whenever she gets the chance, she loves reconnecting with her love for analogue: paper planners and stationery, baking, and sewing.

**Lana Kim, PhD, LMFT** (she/her), was born in Calgary, Alberta, and raised in Vancouver, British Columbia, Canada. She came to the U.S. in the mid-2000s for graduate school and has been practicing for almost 20 years with a special interest in working with couples and parent-child relationships. With a background in medical family therapy, her clinical and research focus includes collaborative care practices, contextual issues in teaching and supervision, relational parenting, and sociocultural and socio-emotional attunement in couple therapy. She regularly provides mentorship to Asian American emerging therapists and as an active member of the American Family Therapy Academy (AFTA) she currently serves as a mentor for their Emerging Leaders in Social Justice fellowship program. She is an associate professor and the program director for the Marriage, Couple, and Family Therapy program at Lewis & Clark College in Portland, Oregon, where she resides with her husband and two children.

**Michael Chen, M.Div,** (he/him), was born and raised in St. Paul, MN, to Taiwanese immigrants. Currently a PhD student (ABD) at Eastern University in Marriage and Family Therapy, he lives in Philadelphia, PA, with his wife, Rachael, two sons Jamison and Silas, and daughter Evelyn. He has been a leader in campus ministry and university chaplaincy for 15 years; in working with several different organizations and congregations, his focus has been on pastoral counseling of individuals and couples through anxiety, addiction, self-esteem, differentiation within family systems, racial identity, and issues surrounding calling and vocation. He holds a certificate in Narrative Focused Trauma Care through the Allender Center at the Seattle School of Theology and Psychology. He is passionate about research and education around issues of race, the impact of collective trauma, and the emergent field of cultural somatics. His desire is to see trauma-informed resources developed through research and the expansion of educational networks for organizations, churches, and the academy. As an Asian American, he hopes his research will contribute to the overall health of individuals and families in the Asian American community in light of growing anti-Asian violence.

**Ulash Thakore-Dunlap, EdD, LMFT** (she/her), was born in London, United Kingdom (UK). She identifies as Asian Indian, and her father was raised in Uganda, Africa, who moved to London, UK, before the expulsions of Asian Indians during the Idi Amin regime, and her mother was born in Burundi (Africa). Ulash lives in San Francisco, California, with her husband and teen son. Her clinical work and private practice focus on supporting Asian and Asian Americans around life transitions, anxiety, racial trauma, and cultural identity. Ulash's research focuses on adolescents, South Asians, school-based mental health, and graduate counseling education. She is assistant professor of school counseling and program coordinator at California State University, East Bay. When not working, Ulash loves family walks along Ocean Beach and hanging out with her friends and family.

**Bowbay Liang-Hua Feng, LMFT** (she/her), was born in Berkeley, California, and spent many years traveling and living internationally. Her father is an immigrant from Taiwan, and her mother came from the Midwest United States (Iowa). She identifies as multiracial, Chinese, German, Norwegian, Irish,

English, and Native American. She brings over 20 years of experience in mindfulness, meditation, spirituality, and martial arts. She incorporates multicultural awareness and issues of diversity in teaching and in her practice as a licensed marriage and family therapist. She co-presented an interactive workshop at the AAMFT-CA Annual Conference regarding working with multi-ethnic and biracial clients and worked as part-time faculty at The Wright Institute, in the masters in counseling program where she mentored and supported students. The majority of her clients are immigrants, or second and third generation, and hold diverse identities. She has a practice built on collaborative self-empowerment and helping people through complex trauma, transitions, relationships, identity development, grief, and quality of life issues. She has a great love for nature and connecting with friends, family, and community.

**Natalie Hsieh, MA, MS, PhD** (she/her), grew up in San Diego, the younger daughter of parents from China and Hong Kong who came to the U.S. as students. She nurtures her Chinese/Asian American identity through relationships with her family of origin, Taiwanese American spouse, their extended families, and several Chinese/Taiwanese/Asian American Christian church families her parents, spouse, and lifelong friends have planted or pastored. Natalie trained in family therapy to enrich her role as a "bridge builder" and mentor of second-generation youth and young adults in Chinese and Taiwanese immigrant churches. Her dissertation research explores themes of relational shame and resilience within the bicultural identity narratives of 1.5 and second-generation Chinese Americans. Natalie holds a PhD in Systems, Families, and Couples, an MS in Marital and Family Therapy (Loma Linda University), an MA in Theological Studies (Bethel Seminary), and an MA in Psychology (Stanford University). She is an assistant professor in clinical counseling at Pt. Loma Nazarene University and is in clinical practice in San Diego, where she lives with her spouse Nick and their son and daughter.

**Wonyoung L. Cho, PhD, LMFT** (she/her), was born in South Korea and moved to the U.S. at the age of nine. She is bilingual and bi-cultural and spent most of her life identifying as a transnational Korean, having struggled with being too Korean for Korean Americans, too American for Koreans, and too Asian for Americans. Currently, she identifies as a 1.5-generation Korean American, and works as an assistant professor in the Marriage Couple and Family Therapy program at Lewis & Clark Graduate School of Education and Counseling in Portland, OR. She is actively involved in the American Family Therapy Academy (AFTA) and Asian American Psychological Association (AAPA). Her work primarily focuses on using multilingualism and translanguaging frameworks to inform culturally responsive and socioculturally attuning pedagogy and practices. Her clinical experiences include working in a multidisciplinary team in a medical setting focusing on children and youth and supervising associates who straddle multiple cultures, languages, and identities.

**Amy Tuttle, PhD, LMFT** (she/her), was born and raised in California's Central Valley. She is biracial, the daughter of her Japanese American mother and white father, and she is Yonsei, a fourth-generation Japanese American. Her professional interests include diversity and sociocultural issues in teaching and clinical work, intervention with marginalized and under-resourced families and communities, relational parenting, clinical supervision, and intergenerational issues of trauma and injustice. She directs the Family Legacy Project, an ongoing qualitative research study examining the intergenerational effects of the incarceration of Japanese Americans during World War II. She is a professor of psychology at Pepperdine University's Graduate School of Education and Psychology, and she currently resides in San Diego with her husband and three children.

## References

Aráullo, K. (2023). The first Asian American settlement established by Filipino fishermen. https://www.history.com/news/first-asian-american-settlement-filipino-st-malo

Budiman, A., & Ruiz, N.G. (2021). Key facts about Asian Americans, a diverse and growing population. https://www.pewresearch.org/short-reads/2021/04/29/key-facts-about-asian-americans/. Retrieved on November 29, 2023.

Hsu, M. Y. (2015). *The good immigrants: How the yellow peril became the model minority*. Princeton University Press. http://www.jstor.org/stable/j.ctt1h4mhst

McDowell, T., Knudson-Martin, C., & Bermudez, J. M. (2019). Third-order thinking in family therapy: Addressing social justice across family therapy practice. *Family Process*, *58*(1), 9–22. https://doi.org/10.1111/famp.12383.

Nadal, K. L. (2019). The Brown Asian American movement: Advocating for South Asian, Southeast Asian, and Filipino American communities. *Asian American Policy Review*, *29*, 2+. https://link.gale.com/apps/doc/A645063413/AONE?u=anon~3e206038&sid=googleScholar&xid=1fb546ac.

Pyke, K. (2000), *"The Normal American Family" as an Interpretive Structure of Family Life Among Grown Children of Korean and Vietnamese Immigrants*. Journal of Marriage and Family, 62: 240-255. https://doi.org/10.1111/j.1741-3737.2000.00240.

Okihiro, G. Y. (2015). *American history unbound: Asians and Pacific Islanders* (1st ed.). University of California Press. http://www.jstor.org/stable/10.1525/j.ctv1wxqh8.

# Part I

# Contextualizing Silence and Invisibility

If you sit with me
  to eat my food
please sit with me
  in my tears
  and suffering too.

To see a body like yours, like mine, brutalized over and over again, then told it was your fault, what were they even doing there, a million more where you came from—but let me eat your food, watch your movies, wear your robes, I'll tell you about my Asian sister-in-law, let me say hello in your language to impress you, let me tell you about the Vietnam War and the Korean War and my time stationed in Japan, let me tell you how much I love kimchi and bulgogi, I love the K-Pop on Jimmy Fallon or was it Kimmel, make me fried rice some day, your English is so good by the way, and your baby daughter has the most interesting eyes, but tell me about your pain and I will tell you it's not real, it happens to everyone anyway, tell us at this panel and Q&A, but we only have half an hour today, you have no history or future or feelings of your own, you are my decoration and my proof of diversity, you are the authority on all eastern culture so tell me your story and pronounce your name but leave out all your hopes and pain.

All I feel is rage.
This grief is only the surface.
I am enraged.
For the love of God,
see us,
hear us.

J.S. Park

J.S. Park [@jspark3000]. (2021, March 17). [Photo of poem by J.S. Park]. Retrieved from //www.instagram.com/p/CMhTxdwhfGg/?utm_source=ig_web _copy_link&igsh=MzRlODBiNWFlZA==

DOI: 10.4324/9781003321590-2

# Chapter 1

# Asian Americans' Invisibilization and Racialization

## Our Transcontextual Journeys

*Saliha Bava*

Juli[1] and Sam sought therapy because Sam wanted to be more "open and vulnerable" as they had just given birth to their first child, Jason. Juli, a second-generation Taiwanese American in her late 30s, ran a boutique design firm. Sam, an African American man in his late 30s, headed up a niche financial consultancy firm.

Varun, a 32-year-old Asian Indian man had immigrated from India to the U.S. for his MBA, called to make an appointment about dating in the U.S. I heard something in his soft voice that I was unable to place. Was it hesitancy, doubt, shyness, and/or shame?

Ifran and Yasmeen, a newlywed couple in their 30s, sought therapy to discuss their financial conflicts. In their late twenties, they identified as Muslim Americans whose parents immigrated from Bangladesh.

\*\*\*

How do we understand culture? Each of the stories sounds like classic couples therapy with cultural issues notably in play. From the cross-cultural marriage of Juli and Sam to Varun's immigrant story of dating to Ifran and Yasmeen's navigation of cultural gender roles, we see culture in play. Do we understand culture as ethnicity or race here? My working assumption is that all couples are in cross-cultural relationships where they are navigating and negotiating their intersectional identities to create their couple identity while navigating multiple contexts. And culture is more than ethnicity or race. Drawing on Celia Falicov's (1996) definition of culture, I view it as a "shared set of world views, meanings, and adaptive behaviors derived from simultaneous membership and participation in a multiplicity of contexts" or social groups that one identifies with (p. 374). Though culture is often used as shorthand for one's identity, it is not one's identity. Rather culture, understood as our collective spoken and unspoken social contracts and arrangements, shapes our identity. This crucial distinction between identity and culture is a key anti-racist practice I adopt in my work as subsequently described.

As a South Asian therapist who has practiced therapy for over 25 years, I'm constantly negotiating and navigating my identity with each of my clients just

DOI: 10.4324/9781003321590-3

as I do in my personal life daily. Not because I am an immigrant in the U.S., but because all conversations are potentially identity-navigating experiences. However, in the U.S., we speak of culture as an othered construct, while not recognizing the culture of whiteness as organizing. The culture of whiteness is one which institutionally and socially upholds the supremacy of whiteness even as it obscures itself while racializing Blackness, thus, making itself the norm. It ranges from "white people's conviction of their natural superiority" (Morrison in Harris, 2020, p. 5) to "white is might," "white is right," and "white is most beautiful" while denigrating all that is not white. These socially constructed racialized values are systemically, structurally, and discursively maintained by people of varying racial identities, not limited to white people. By actively adopting an anti-Blackness stance, whiteness sets up a divisive system of binaries and positions power into hierarchies (Harris, 2020) with immigrant groups seeking the access that whiteness affords. Thus, the global majority immigrants who are not Black or white often experience the inherent invisibilization and marginalization of racialized U.S. where, due to slavery and colonization, race is seen as property (Harris, 2020) and denied simultaneously.[2]

In this chapter, I unpack the invisibilization of Asian Americans[3] as the interplay of racial binaries and intersectional invisibility. Drawing on multiple contexts, I unpack the *discursive*—the play of language, meaning-making, and the interplay of the social and relational—to illustrate the reification of the social systemic discourses of who counts and why. These discourses both shape and are shaped by the structural arrangements of how race and immigration are organized in the U.S. Additionally, the U.S.'s standing as a global leader in knowledge-based economies mediates migration while obscuring its racialized immigration processes. Adopting a socio-relational perspective, I unpack the positionality of Asian Americans and their invisibilization that is maintained by the myths of model minority, the perpetual foreigner, the tech-savvy yet passive foreigner who is dehumanized as lacking emotions and individuality. All of these myths are compounded by the myth of cultural homogeneity that obscures the linguistic, cultural, religious, national/regional, and immigrant diversities (Sue et al., 2021; Yip et al., 2021).

Consequently, in my practice I have grappled with how to explore racial invisibilization and reductive homogeneity by zooming in and out of context. In a parallel way, I also grapple with the complexity and contradictions I experience as a racialized being navigating my own racial and social conscientization processes across overlapping contexts. Navigating these complexities and contradictions in clinical practices within the U.S. led me to craft the following three relational dialogic resources, described later—*shared inquiry of cultural curiosity, the relational discursive loop,* and *hyperlinked identities and conversations.* Drawing on these resources, I conclude with illustrations of how to counteract invisibilization and racialization by engaging in *transcontextual* (Bateson, 2023) conversations to host client's sense-making. Though I will be speaking as an Asian-identifying therapist by drawing on my therapeutic work with Asians/Asian Americans, these relational resources can be adapted based on the varying positionalities of the conversational partners. This chapter is written from the voice of an intersectional, transnational, Asian woman in an interracial marriage with a white American man, living in the U.S. for 25+ years while holding an Indian passport.

## Unpacking Dominance: Racialization of Asian Americans

Speaking about dominance as the umbrella category by which to speak of racism is a double-edged sword. Shereen Daniels (2022), a Human Resource Strategist, cautions us that to speak of racism in terms of anti-dominance rather than as anti-racism is to speak in terms of a generalist and will not lead to specific interventions (p. 151). Speaking of dominance obscures the specificities of racism. However, to not speak of the interlocking systems of dominance risks stripping away complexity and intersectionality. Audre Lorde (2020) reminds us that "we do not live single-issue lives" (p. 133) and to talk of our lives as such is one of the hallmarks of any dominance-based system. Racialization—a socio-political process of ascribing racial identity—is a contested term. It arises not just from the process of racism but also from multiple contexts (e.g., economic, political, colonial, social, interpersonal, etc.), overlapping and defining each other. Thus, I speak of racism from an intersectional perspective (Crenshaw, 1991) acknowledging systemic thinker Nora Bateson's (2023) notion of *transcontextuality*—the overlap of multiple contexts that form a complex system. This does not preclude specific anti-racist interventions, which as Daniels notes are crucial. What it does is help us notice dominance as organizing across a range of interacting contexts creating complex interlocking systems, as is with Asian American lives. I invite you to notice how racism mediates and is mediated by multiple contexts as well as held up, reproduced, reorganized, or troubled and potentially dismantled by our critically reflexive participation.

Black people and their histories have been largely absent and legislatively continue to be obscured in the name of banning critical race theory (CRT). As comedian Roy Wood, Jr. powerfully states, "anti-CRT policies are an attack on Black history and an attempt to erase the contributions of Black people from the history books" (C-SPAN, 2023, time 1:20:33). And this invisibilization of history extends to how we talk of race in the U.S.—in black and white ways. No pun intended. Decontextualized, the binary construction of race is not only the game of white supremacy but also the extended game of invisibilization of Asian Americans and their histories. Not only are Blacks written out, but so are all other cultures of color that are not white. Racial subjugation stems from the following processes of domination:

- **Binary constructions:** The U.S. construction of the Black and white binary structure of racism predicates the absence of other "races" and forms of racism even as it creates the construct of race and racism (Gines, 2013; Westmoreland, 2013). By creating an *us vs them* context, it wipes out plurality to aid in the creation of the supremacy of the singular, dominant voice. It not only obscures non-Blacks who are not white but also racism against them by its binary construction. This binary construction keeps anti-Asian racism out of the anti-Black racist discourses (Westmoreland, 2013) and positions non-whites who are not Black as outsiders. So, the challenge is how do we conceptualize anti-blackness *in relationship to* other forms of racial violence (nativism, xenophobia, etc.) without the making of binary? How do we not split intersectional identities (which is another device of domination)? Drawing on Bateson's (2023) call for transcontextual descriptions, I orient to a way to go beyond the binary call by noticing the relational processes in the making of the construct of Asian American identities.
- **Essentialization:** A binary construction of racism is compounded by essentializing of everything else that is "other," including the telling of a single story of racism. Although Black identity like Asian identity is heterogeneous, it is constructed as a monolithic group. Speaking in terms of "sameness" of experiences erases the plurality and conflicting stories of our experiences (Badwall, 2016). It also results in the essentialization of that which is considered superior, enforcing narrow definitions of what is allowed even for folks who are part of the dominant groups. For example, the effeminate portrayal of Asian American men in popular culture compared to their hypermasculine white American counterparts (Fischer & Seidman, 2016, p. 55). Essentializing is a form of discursive practice, where in talk and text we further racism. Thus, whiteness is maintained by othering all other stories and homogenizing diverse stories of subordinate groups as a single story without any nuance, e.g., seeing all non-whites as BIPOCs.
- **Intersectional Invisibility:** Racial understandings are constructs of single-issue analysis within the U.S. For instance, women of color stories are relegated to either "woman" or "person of color," obscuring intersectionality (Crenshaw, 1991). Consequently, dominant systems achieve control over intertwining multiplicities by obscuring intersectionality. Intersectional understandings are transcontextual. These complicate and break down the making of single stories. Thus, understanding identities as plural, including the contradictions, is very much needed for unpacking complex Asian American lives.
- **Coloniality:** The twentieth century saw most of the Asian world colonized by Europe. And it lives on as coloniality—an unfinished project[4]

post-independence showing up in social, professional, and knowledge-making practices (Badwall, 2016). Walter Mignolo (2021) states "racism is the outcome of the colonial difference—the technology to inflict colonial wounds" (p. 144). How does colonization continue to operate in our everyday practices? How and who are contesting, re-producing, and re-signifying the racialized therapeutic discourses that shape our materialized lives? Contextually unpacking historical and current forms of coloniality, especially in terms of knowledge, expertise, and professional practices, is foundational to therapeutic engagement of Asian Americans, especially if one seeks to adopt an anti-colonial or de-colonial stance in therapy.

All of the above contribute to racial invisibilization and prevent interracial solidarity (Yancy & Kim, 2015). And the same holds true for Asian American racialization which emerges in the relationships across contexts that create and maintain a culture of white supremacy.

### Invisibilization of Asian Americans: In Relationship with Relationships

The pan-ethnic term "Asian American" coined in 1968 by UC Berkeley student activists Emma Gee and Yuji Ichiokato (Zhou, 2021) is a quintessential example of the power of the discursive. This historical term created to organize the political power for Asians in the U.S. obscures not only the socio-cultural and historical diversity but also the health, economic, educational, and social disparities often replicating the inequities of their country of origin. Nearly all (90%) Asian adults living in the U.S. report more within-group cultural differences than commonalities though six-in-ten report feeling connected to what happens to other Asian Americans (Ruiz et al., 2023). Asian Americans frequently face invisibility because of their perceived "model minority" status which "invites a kind of political affiliation with whiteness" (Yancy & Kim, 2015, para 27). This stereotype assumes that all Asian Americans are successful and high achieving, which can lead to the erasure of their diverse experiences and challenges. Such racial tropes exploit Asian stereotypes to benefit white supremacy, by obscuring social processes, homogenizing Asian diversity, and invisibilizing the inequity gaps among Asians in the U.S.

Lee and Zhou's (2015) research shows how institutional elements interface with historical and cultural factors granting advantages to certain Asian American groups, thus creating an achievement paradox for other Asian Americans who do not "succeed" accordingly. This compounds invisibility with a sense of failure and lack of belonging with one's own. Social discourses obscure the 1965 U.S. immigration reform that privileged selecting highly educated and skilled immigrants[5] while perpetuating the myth of Asians' obsession with scholastic achievement (Lee & Zhou, 2015). Yet, despite these high-status granting practices and stereotypes curated by our institutional, historical, and social processes, there continues to be a lack of representation of Asian Americans in sciences (Yip et al., 2021), media, and politics which further invisibilizes them in society.

People with multiple marginalized identities (e.g., Asian American Muslim gay man) may experience *intersectional invisibility* (Purdie-Vaughns & Eibach, 2008), leading to feelings of overcompensation, isolation, and alienation. This can include historical, cultural, political, and legal invisibilities that are sourced from the ideological prototypes/stereotypes of the respective referential social groups. And such invisibilizing extends to our professional lives where those who seek to study Asian Americans do so at risk to their careers and are advised not to take it up (Lee & Zhou, 2015; Yip et al., 2021). I have seen this take the form of Asian American trainees not wanting to see clients of their ethnicity so as not to be pigeonholed. Or becoming the enforcers of the model minority myth with their clients when parents are struggling with their child's school performance. These are all ways to be in relationship with relationships to our social stories that seek to invisibilize us.

### Deconstructing the Colonial Project in Asia

Of the Asian Americans in the U.S., about 54% are first-generation immigrants, 34% are U.S.-born children of immigrant parents, and 14% are third or higher generation (Ruiz et al., 2023). An Asian American life is an entanglement of many Western threads woven into the social fabric of what we bracket as Asians in the U.S. We all bring our stories of our lands and family migration legacies. To understand our identity stories is to understand the colonial histories of the lands we arrived from, bringing varying narratives of superiority and subjugation.

Kohn and Reddy (2023) characterize the *colonial project* as a systematic political and military domination, settlement, and economic and sovereignty control of lands by European nations for their own economic and strategic interests. By the end of the 19th century, Europe and the U.S. had divided almost the entire world, except for Japan and China. While Japan and the U.S. joined the forces of colonization, the different European powers weakened China with their controlling interests. World Wars I and II stressed the European economies and the rising local freedom movements forced their hand for independence. The 1940s to 1960s saw "more than fifty new sovereign nations emerge from imperial domination" (TimeMaps, n.d.). This historical context creates complex material realities for families, including our clients and us. The only way to unpack its impact is to learn how these stories have traveled and uniquely shaped various intergenerational family stories and migration legacies, at times making these connections in therapy and supervision. Stories of survival ranging from allegiance to imperial powers to freedom fighters exist in varying forms within

Asian family legacies. These historical stories travel as culture, traditions, and mores. They become family stories. They take on the relational and emotional forms of silence, pride, perfection, control, shame, navigations, negotiations, adaptations, messiness, contradictions, connection, loss, anxiety, sadness, joy, audacity, resistance, returning, discovery, and much more. They are organizing even as they remain invisible and invisibilizing.

My own journey has been to piecemeal my cultural stories as I engage and listen to my family's stories. Yet I am far from having forged my story fully; it will remain incomplete and unfinished yet felt as the previous generations echo in me (Menakem, 2017). I grew up being told my grandfathers were overseas traders who were Rowthers—my paternal grandfather's last name and the term for Tamil-speaking Muslim community who were occupationally traders. In exploring the history of Rowthers, I discovered that I am the granddaughter of the traders who traveled the "spice routes" (the Maritime Silk Roads) from Southern India to Malacca, current day Malaysia and Singapore. But for how many generations and how they came to be traveling the international trade routes was left untold as we stayed close to our two-generational story of business loss for both of my grandfathers. The loss of business created a cloud of economic and ambiguous loss which shapes our current day family narrative. Even as we turn away from business and family business stories, I sense the enduring pride of belonging to the Rowthers/traders. This contradiction grew my conviction to own my business self, even as the immediate family message was one of prohibition. Learning to live within this contradiction was echoed by my postmodern education to embrace rather than resolve contradictions. Postmodernism, my theoretical home (Bava, 2019, 2022a), became my way to dance with these contradictions.

We grow our current worlds, remaking our past, by seeing and seeking our place in the imagined futures. We become through our discursive practices of interactions, words, stories, artifacts, and mores that we bring forth. The therapeutic context goes on to become one such space where through conversations we become our future selves borne from our search for dignity, connection, and meaning. As therapists, our responsiveness to the client's search invites us to maintain curiosity by bringing forth a sensitivity to the histories and contexts that travel through the generational stories to the current relationships and spaces they call home.

As systemic therapists, we explore stories of pain and pride (Sheinberg & Fraenkel, 2000). Most Asians carry the colonial project (Kohn & Reddy, 2023) with us as we or our forebears arrived in the U.S. The colonial project, a source of pain for many, can also be a source of pride or contradiction for other Asians. For instance, my parents made life choices to provide their daughters with a good education, which included English medium education hosted by a Catholic school. Consequently, English education, a vestige of colonialism, affords me a ride to the U.S. Thus, we have to hold such contradictions with curiosity even as we explore the interplay of the colonial project in the present world. The therapeutic space becomes one of the spaces to explore these entanglements and contradictions of our histories which become the present-day storied lives we live.

### Who Counts as "Asian" in Asian American

I have not felt seen as an "Asian" in the U.S. Lee and Ramakrishnan (2020) drawing on the 2016 National Asian American Survey state "the default for Asian is still East Asian" (p. 1751). So, being invited to write this opening chapter is a process of standing up to the socio-political-legal narrative that splits us Asians in terms of who counts as Asian. Harpalani (2013) states South Asians in the U.S. experience "racial ambiguity—the changing racial characterization of a person or group, depending on the local and historical context" (p. 83).

The term Asian in the U.S. is constructed racially rather than geographically representing the racial construction of our identities. Geographically, the Asian identity would extend to West Asia with Turkey being the westernmost state (see Figure 1.1). Until the Immigration and Nationality Act of 1952, "fighting for the White racial designation was an imperative step to obtain the full right of citizenship" (Awad et al., 2021, p. 116). Lee and Ramakrishnan (2020) note that,

> racial assignment is a multipronged, potentially fraught process that involves how governments define racial categories and assign groups to those categories, how immigrant and national origin groups understand and assign themselves into racial categories, and how out-groups understand and assign immigrant and national origin groups to the same racial categories.
>
> (p. 5)

The U.S.'s racial discourses combined with its status as an economic leader whose currency defines the global market and the Western world's positioning of the U.S. as the world leader with military power shapes how immigrants are granted not only citizenship but also racial and ethnic status. The terms *Far-East* Asia referring to East Asia, *Middle East* referring to West Asia, and *Near East* referring to Central Asia are all terms that privilege the Western vantage point of view (Coman, 2019). People of these regions do not refer to themselves as "Far-East" or "Middle East." These language practices of the West and the corresponding discourses are not limited to shaping census data but have very real material effects on how people are received and positioned in everyday interactions making them further visible or invisible. Lee and Ramakrishnan (2020) illustrate that "while Indians and Pakistanis racially assign themselves as Asian, they are not assigned as such by other Asian groups" (p. 13). This is the play of the discursive. It illustrates the collective social positioning of identities that occurs in language, text, interaction, and meaning. What is played up is a reified

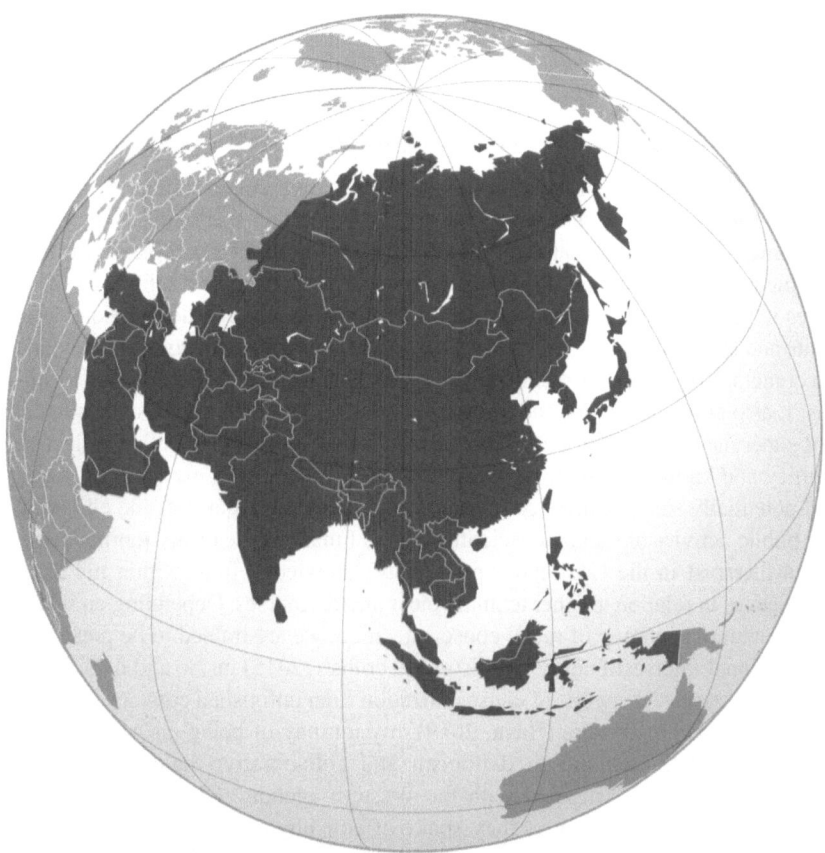

*Figure 1.1* Orthographic projection of Asia (image from: Koyos + Ssolbergj, CC BY-SA 4.0, via Wikimedia Commons)

systemic discourse of who counts and how via the process of racialization of immigration.

Thus, the construction of an Asian in the U.S. is based on race rather than a geographical location. This racial discourse in the U.S. is *internalized* by East Asian groups to maintain its privileged position as the default Asian excluding South Asians with no mention of West Asians who are referred to as Middle Eastern. *Is this splitting of Asia not a Western power play that we as Asians play into?* For instance, geographically, the Asian population, which is 12.66 times the North American population, is equivalent to 59.76% of the total world population at 4.752 billion people (Worldometers) compared to the North American population of 375 million people which is 4.73% of the world population. *How does it change the conversation to own our collective power in naming ourselves and reclaiming "Asian"?*

## Dialogic Resources for Orienting Socio-Relationally

The ethical call of our practice is to host consultative conversations that orient toward dignity, respect, and equity such that people feel seen and heard within the context of cultural dynamism. Given the above-described complexity, I have grappled with the question of how one explores the transcontextuality of experiences in the therapeutic setting without reproducing systems of domination? Like white and Black therapists, our "work" is not done before we engage in therapeutic encounters. The nature of racialization is such that it is not limited to our identities, it also colors our work and knowledge-making practices such as our clinical and supervisory conversations. This chapter, a case in point, is both a reflective journey and knowledge-making. Even as I write, I'm shaping my identity stories and potentially shaping practice (culture). Written at the request of the editors, it is a public activity of racial conscientization as I make sense of my journey as an Asian therapist in the U.S., thus "producing" knowledge from within my lived experiences in relation to other textual voices and discourses. Depending on where we are with our journey of racial conscientization, we are trained to be present to our relational intersectionality (Addison & Coolhart, 2015) inside and outside our clinical practice as the work of conscientization is an unfinished conversation.

As described elsewhere (Bava, 2019), my journey of being an Asian immigrant in the U.S. led me to dialogism and collaborative-dialogic practices (Anderson, 2022). I struggled with the Western agenda of individualism that kept us entity-focused even as they spoke of empathy and compassion. A neoliberal agenda which repositions "social issues…as individual attributes" (Klein & Mills, 2017, p. 2001) and where culture and race are constructed as static rather than dynamic interplays of social processes by which we are positioned. Neoliberalism, a form of financial ideology that promotes individualism, simultaneously feeds us insecurities and remedies as part of the global psychologically centered practices that shape well-being and therapeutics (Hardy & Ness, 2015; Sullum, 2020). U.S.'s historical, colonial, and racial processes are foundational to the neoliberal marketplace (the current-day colonial capitalism). It was this initially unnamable, troubling orientation toward human social nature that led me to relational responsiveness (Anderson, 2012; Bava, 2022a; Shotter, 2015a, 2015b, 2016) and social responsiveness—positively generative dialogic resources (Gergen, 2023).

Drawing on social constructionism (Anderson, 2022; Gergen, 2023), *relational responsiveness* is a reflexive way of orienting to the process of **making meaning together from within the spontaneous flow of our experiences and interactions** locally. *Social responsiveness* is a reflexive way of orienting to the process of **making meaning together from within our social stories and structures**. *Reflexivity* refers to the situated and constitutive nature of such responsivity, noticing the relationships that shape relationships. Relational and social responsiveness are recursively interlinked as illustrated in Figure 1.2. McNamee (2008) highlights that such responsiveness is situated or contextualized by our historical, social, cultural, relational processes, and local expectations and repertoires. I offer three dialogic resources for transcontextually attuning to the *generative interplay of relational responsiveness* and *the social complexity* within clinical spaces and beyond. These resources grew out of my relational efforts to make sense as I navigated clinical and supervisory worlds as an Asian in the U.S. They offer a window into my praxis, and I invite you, the reader, to reflect on your sense-making processes and contribute to how might we conceptualize our positionalities from *within* our practices and vice versa.

### Shared Inquiry as Cultural Curiosity: Attuned Listening

*Cultural curiosity* is a process of shared inquiry to unpack the cultural discourses that shape our identity and how we continue to act back on the cultural stories to claim our preferred identity performances. Harlene Anderson (2022) defines *shared inquiry* as a way of being and becoming where we engage in mutual exploration of what and how the client tells their story.

Juli and Sam set the tone for therapy by seeking to focus on Sam and his quest for vulnerability. I was curious what it meant for him and how things might be different if he performed greater vulnerability. I also wondered how vulnerability might be tied to structural violence. He focused on his years growing up as a kid taking care of his parents who were physically present but emotionally absent due to alcohol use. He had to take care of his siblings as the eldest and as an eight-year-old; when his parents failed to come through for him, he promised himself to never land himself or his children where they would get hurt or want for anything. While the latter turned into making money, the hurt transformed into not being vulnerable.

Adopting a culturally curious stance with Juli and Sam unfolded as a shared inquiry of various contexts including his family culture and the culture of the places where he grew up. While we attuned to the intersectionalities within his identity stories, we also attended to interplay with Juli's stories of intersecting identities. Over the weeks, we explored how familial and social stories had shaped their relationship to emotional expression and the notion of vulnerability. Starting with Sam's story of how he had decided to shut down all his expectations and feelings while only focusing on getting on with his efforts to make a good life, we came to explore his context-dependent intersecting identity performances. Though Sam briefly spoke of being a Black man in the U.S., he focused more on the emotional neglect rather than how his racial or gender identity shaped him. Meanwhile, Juli spoke of being second-generation Taiwanese

American and raised in an affluent business family. She reflected on how her family was particular about her educational choices as they wanted her to pursue a business degree and follow the family business even though she was interested in the creative arts. While I was aware of being an Asian woman like Juli, I did not assume a commonness because of differences in our ethnicity, immigrant status, socio-economic histories, age, and more. And, with Sam, though we were both brown-skinned, I was aware of how my Indian identity mediates my experiences in the U.S. compared to that of an African American man. Attuning to the socio-cultural context (McDowell et al., 2022) and the circulating conversations of our times, and drawing on our rich intersectional conversations, I chose to name the presence of racio-ethnicity in our lives and how it operates differently for each of us. And, seeking their permission, I wondered aloud how it organized their lives and more specifically, their way of performing vulnerability. Sam responded that at work he does not show "any weakness" as a Black man, so no one will question his business decisions. And Juli spoke of how their financial status mediates her Asian status.

Thus, a transcontextual focus of our clinical conversations was an exploration of the interplay of culture and identity (Bava & Greene, 2023) even as we attended to the interplay of the therapist and client's social locations. I spoke of culture as "the water we make together even as we are swimming in it." We *created a distinction between culture and identity by leaning into our mutual cultural curiosity* of how they navigated their received familial and cultural stories as they defined and negotiated their performances of relating that shaped their identity stories. Such *curiosity is infectious and invitational*. Sam and Juli would arrive with new stories from their childhood or an everyday story of how they were aware of their identity. For instance, once they opened up a session reflecting on a weekend incident and noticing how they walked down the sidewalk as they weaved through other people, either making space or taking-up space. I leaned into curiosity, uncertain where it might lead, as we engaged these stories to unpack culture and identity in the process of making sense of their relationship to vulnerability, the initial goal for therapy.

A shared inquiry is one where we adopt a *not-knowing* stance (Anderson, 2012, 2022) that generates curiosity as we engage in understanding the other's culture even as we reflect together in the making of culture itself. We do so by engaging in what Anderson (2022) refers to as speaking to listen. It is a way of being responsive where we do not bring a pre-understanding to our questions; where speaking, listening, hearing, responding, and understanding all go hand-in-hand (Anderson, 2022, p. 14). As I engaged with Juli and Sam, even as I stayed aware of the intertwining threads of racial and ethnic identities, I did not bring a pre-understanding of how these particular identities might have shaped their vulnerability. I was listening to understand how stories of identity and culture interwove as they spoke of vulnerability, while staying curious as they spoke of intersecting invisible or less known identities. I was listening to what was important for them and what they left out from their storylines. I was listening to how their story not only moved me but more so moved them (Andersen, 1996).

We are listening not only to what is said but also engaging in what John Shotter refers to as "attuned listening," an *engaged activity of meaning-making*. He describes it as

> listening in a way in which we are oriented wholly towards the otherness of the other – entails letting their speech *flow through us*, so to speak, to such an extent that it 'moves' us, that it generates movements of feeling within us that will, at first, more likely than not make no sense to us; we are confused, bewildered, we do not yet know 'our way about'; however, if we 'dwell in' it for a while, and begin to 'move around' within it, a 'something', an 'it' begins to emerge.
>
> (2015a, p, 10)

Shotter cautions us against listening in ways where we seek to take up the other's content (what is said) and assimilate it with what is familiar to us, such that we fail to see the other. Instead of attending to the "patterns of already spoken words" he invites us into *a way of relating where the other happens to us*. As Sam and Juli spoke of vulnerability, my thoughts briefly traveled to Brene Brown's work on vulnerability, seeking to assimilate what they were speaking with what was familiar to me from the cultural ethos of our times. I caught myself and instead shifted my sensibility toward my body, seeking to understand from within their stories allowing it to *flow through me* and be moved.

Such a way of engaging cultural curiosity moves us beyond cultural competency of knowing what is cultural (or vulnerability, in this case) for the other and instead moves us into a relational space of shared, mutual inquiry where we experience the other. It is what Marsha McDonough speaks of as *heartfelt curiosity* which is "a fundamental practice for tapping into the common humanity in a conversational partnership or shared inquiry" (2022, p. 77). Cultural curiosity without heartfelt curiosity can become cultural competency in the form of fitting people into cultural categories. Laura Brown (2009) critiques the popular view of cultural competence which "is about *them*—it's about the Other, the client who is diverse, and about how to address the problem of dealing with that Other in psychotherapy" (p. 342). Such a view originates from psychotherapy practices developed from, for, and by the whiteness gaze that continues othering the racialized other resulting in "the acquisition of data and algorithms about various groups of people" (Brown, 2009, p. 342). Instead, we drop from the head into the felt movement arising from within the interactive moment where the emergent meaning is formed and transformed in the engagement *with* the other who is shaping us.

So, how might we engage and track conversations with our clients to unpack the interplay of culture and identity, given the complexity of our intersectional identities, relational intersectionalities, and emergent meanings?

### The Relational Discursive Loop: Relational and Social Responsiveness

Our language is not mirroring reality, rather, in language, meaning is jointly constructed by the participants who are relationally, socially, and historically situated (Anderson, 2012, 2022). Mikhail Bakhtin (1981) reminds us, our stories are not exclusively ours; "it is the *product of the interaction of the interlocutors*, and broadly speaking, the product of the whole complex *social situation* in which it has occurred" (p. 30). In language, people craft their unique identity stories from within the invisible web of relationships and conversations which is part of the rich transcontextual backdrop. *Relationships shaping relationships*. Thus, engaging in a shared inquiry with heartfelt curiosity and attuned listening we stay open to how the words, phrases, and conversations touch us. We build on the curiosity of what is contextual and/or emergent.

Yet, in my practice, both as a therapist and trainer, I grappled with how to attend to that which is *invisible yet deeply felt*. How do we get curious about the complex social situation that is being invoked even as it remains unnamed at times? How do we get curious about the stories that invisibly might be guiding the multiple (con)textual nature of our felt conversations? The systemic view, drawing on the onion model, offers a visualization of multiple systems that locates the person in the center and the social and cultural as the outer circles in a concentric diagram. However, it fails to bring forth the interplay of the social and interactional. Growing up in India, I did not experience the social as separate from everyday interactions. I needed a visualization that hosted the co-constitutive nature of the social and the everyday interactions. Thus, I drew on Bakhtin to craft the *relational discursive loop*[6] (Bava, 2022b) to explore *words as windows into worlds—social discourses*; an interplay of the relational and social responsiveness. To make "visible" that which is invisible, we engage *the relational discursive loop as a navigational guide* of the interplay from the somatic to the social.

The Relational Discursive Loop helps us to see how our somatic experiences, utterances, and interactions are recursively intertwined with the structural and systemic processes which in turn are shaped and shape our storied realities (Figure 1.2).

A. **Somatic Sensory:** Our bodies are somatically responsive to our everyday experiences. These somatic experiences are shaped and in turn shape our words, actions, and interpretations.

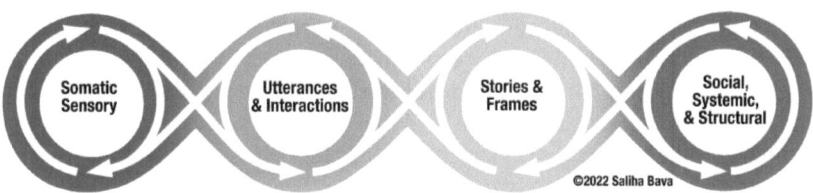

*Figure 1.2* Relational discursive loop

B. **Utterances and Interactions:** Through utterances and interactions we are making meaning with others. Our words and interactions simultaneously shape and are shaped by our understandings. We improvise spontaneously, as we calibrate to each other's expressions making micro-adjustments with our words and gestures (nods, smiles, eyes hands, etc.) to coordinate and create shared meanings. The interplay of the somatic and the interactions is understood/interpreted from within the emerging frames of meanings that are negotiated and coordinated within the relational and social context.

C. **Stories/Frames:** The frames and stories are interpretations, that is, socio-relational emergence. In relationships, we negotiate and navigate the situated meanings thus creating local shared meanings which are also being informed by multiple, overlapping contexts. Our interpretations and meanings also emerge from navigating the socially, culturally, and historically situated narratives that are invisible frames for sense-making. These larger frames, often called received scripts, travel as "how things are" or "ought to be done."

D. **Social, Systemic, Structural:** The social, systemic, and structural sedimentations are dynamics that emerged with time from within the engaged dialogic communal processes. Thus, over time they emerge as context both influencing and influenced by our frames, stories, and meanings.

When Varun spoke of the women he was dating, his utterances carried the richness of the large social context. He would often describe a woman as being "out of his league" (utterances) which to me denoted class (social/structural systems), but I remained curious about what he meant by "league." He would go on to refer to her way of dressing and carrying herself, often referring to a distinction made in India between people from a rural part of India as compared to an urban part of India (stories/frames). I was sensitive to how language and dressing, as discursive practices and performances of class, also potentially carried a somatic presence. As a newly arrived immigrant, with limited financial resources, I too had felt physically conscious of my dressing in my efforts to fit into the Western traditions of professionalism. That consciousness, reclaimed as my Indian expression, resistance, and celebration, is still present today. Varun had grown up in a village and through educational achievements had acquired occupational and economic resources that afforded him social status, yet he often described interactions that left him feeling inadequate, stating he had not transcended to the social status accorded to people born into such a class, echoing the caste system that undergirds the Indian social makeup. *Words are windows into worlds.* Varun's stories carried the contradictions of not being man enough as a person of color in the U.S. and not good enough by Indian rural/urban class standards even though he had achieved educational and occupational status; presence of multiple overlapping contexts. As an urban Indian, I too carried the consciousness he spoke of, affording me a shared cultural resource by which to trouble the transitory and the sedimented materializations of his utterances while acknowledging our relational intersectionalities (Addison & Coolhart, 2015).

The relational discursive loop brings forth the recursive interplay between relational and social responsiveness. It helps us to make visible the sedimented social and structural parts of our lives while noticing the dynamism present in producing, reproducing (*"this is how we do it"*), troubling (*"according to whom"*), resisting (*"I choose not to"*), challenging (*"that is outdated"*), and/or dismantling (*"not anymore"*) them. And the dynamism, irrespective of whether we keep alive the social scripts or take them apart, lies in our everyday interactions which underscore our relational agency—actions originating from within the relationships that connect.

### Hyperlinked Conversations and Identities: Navigating Transcontextuality

Sense-making conversations, especially those relating to emerging understandings of one's identities as related to multiple overlapping cultures, are rarely linear. I find these conversations as walking a labyrinth, yet not so patterned, more meandering. More often they are like traversing the internet as we jump from one hyperlink to another. Drawing on my dissertation research, I came to call such dialogues *hyperlinked conversations* (Bava, 2019). The notion of hyperlinked helped me to orient, engage, and become curious *with* our conversational partners about the emerging relationships within their intersectional identity stories which developed as they moved in hyperlinked ways through their stories of identity, context (including culture), and meaning. Hyperlinked conversations help us to navigate multiple contexts to develop transcontextual descriptions that offer possibilities for living while resisting binary, divisive, essentializing stories that insidiously continue the power of colonization and invisibilization. The notion of hyperlinking is my way of owning my heritage to embrace complexity while resisting the notion of story as having a beginning, middle, and an end—the linear narrativization of sense-making. Many stories I grew up with were not so linear. Clinically, I have come to refer hyperlinking as *mutually learning and engaging with how people are connecting "the dots" between their various contextualized identity stories while resisting the urge to essentialize or slot people's stories into predetermined theoretical categories.*[7] By listening for what matters to them and how they seek to make sense, I can host and open up space for us to jump across socio-cultural, historical, political, and many other contexts while concurrently attending to the somatic and emergent meaning.

Ifran and Yasmeen explored their identities of being second-generation Asian Americans as we engaged in a shared inquiry of their received social scripts of marriage, gender roles, work, and more. We hyperlinked to tension and conflict and back to gender relations to living racialized lives in the U.S. Their stories effortlessly wove the various contexts of ethnicity, religion, gender, and immigration with belonging, desire, family, and communication, and much more. I sought to not essentialize or "segregate" their ethnicity stories from the other identity stories as we traversed their complex racialized lives as illustrated below.

*SB:* I wonder how do your parents or your side of the family see your marriage or Yasmeen?

*Ifran:* Well, they think we are young. And tell us we need to settle down and start a family.

*SB:* And you?

*Ifran:* What?

*SB:* Start a family?

*Ifran:* Yes, at some point, but I don't want to change what we have.

*SB:* Like what? (*Seeking a richer understanding*)

*Ifran:* Traveling, going out with friends, trips, being independent, having a good time. My parents didn't do these things. All our trips were to visit family, not going places and seeing the world. I want my children to see the world. (Yasmeen nods)

*SB:* Wow! I see you both feel very strongly about that (*responding to how animated they both sounded and looked*).

*Yasmeen:* Yes, that is what brought us together. We like to travel.

*SB:* What is it about traveling? Does it fit to go down that road? (*Seeking permission, as I was being spontaneously responsive in **hyperlinking to an intersectional identity space** by jumping to another conversational thread while wondering how it might all be contextually interlinked.*)

Clients through their interlinked stories orient us to the conversations that matter or offer a sense of where we might go next which Shotter (2015b) refers to as *action guiding anticipations*. Yasmeen and Ifran's expressions served as an action guiding anticipation of where we might go next. Though I imagined understanding the value of traveling might be a resourceful thread, I sought permission.

*Yasmeen:* Sure. Travel keeps it real.

*SB:* Meaning?

*Yasmeen:* Seeing the world opens the world. You see how you can be, seeing how others live their lives.

*Ifran:* We love to travel and stay with the locals. We want to meet people, talk and hang out. Soak it all up.

*SB:* So, you don't play tourists but seek a more local experience?

*Yasmeen:* ya, but we do go see touristy places.... But it is the people and their stories we love to connect.

*SB:* I think I get the difference, and may I ask what about it compels you?

*Yasmeen:* I love people, but I think more so it reminds us about being us...

*SB:* meaning...

*Yasmeen:* Well, growing up as a Muslim girl here was hard...not to say some of my cousins back home don't have it harder. We had a lot of good stuff, but I was always an outsider. Kind of odd and didn't fit in. For a long time, there was no one who looked like me. Most kids were white. I knew I was not one of them, as my parents were not from here and I didn't get to hang out with them after school stuff. It was school and home. Later, there were a couple of brown kids, but they spoke Spanish and I didn't....so no one really... until I went to high school in NYC which was a big shock. Like the whole world was right there! And, then college was fun, lots of people doing their own thing and I met Ifran, and we would hang out with folks who were all from different parts of the world. It just felt real...you know...we were all different, but we got each other. (*I heard it as immigrant speech for same but different. I curiously made note of the subtextual interplay of racial binaries and intersectional invisibility woven in her transcontextual story.*)

*SB:* So, was that the start of traveling the world? (*Discursive loop choice point: I make a note to later return to the intersectional invisibility and social marginalization **as I read her words** signaling to the structural presence. There are other ways to make sense.*)

*Ifran:* No, not for me. My parents moved to the UK for some time to be with their relatives and then moved back to the U.S. And we went to visit our relatives every Summer. (*Discursive loop note to self: the transcontextuality of movement, access, family relations, support, connection, class, and access.*)

*Yasmeen:* Yes, after we got married, we really started to travel more. My parents didn't travel much because money was tight.

*SB:* So, travel appears to have taken on a different meaning for each of you compared to your parents.

Orienting to their guidance, seeking to understand their situated identity stories as hyperlinked stories or textual spaces, underscores the client's expertise and ways of knowing and becoming (Anderson, 2012, 2022). Attending to our therapeutic conversations as hyperlinked conversations allows for the practice of orienting to the intersectionalities and interconnectedness of our racialized identities. That is why hyperlinked identities and conversations go hand-in-hand. The primary orientation of hyperlinked conversations is attuning to trans-contextuality—multiple overlapping contexts (Bateson, 2023) to host plural intersectional identity stories. Such orienting conversations can help us decenter our positional power in therapy while attending to the circulating social power that mediates our therapeutic conversations.

## Conclusion: A Reflective Invitation

We are living in a neoliberal world (Bhatia & Priya, 2018; Sugarman, 2015) driven by greed-based capitalist politics, where our intersectionally fluid, emergent, plural identities (Bava, 2019) are reductionistically profiled into thin storylines. In such a world, the culturally racialized politics reduced to divisive identity politics strips us of our rich, thick, contradictory stories. In reclaiming our contradictions while resisting being stripped down to single identity discourses, as Asian American, we reclaim our complex heritages and counter the U.S.'s racialized binary and invisiblizing discourses.

To counter these problematic subjugating narratives, I suggest we unpack the interplay of culture and identity. Navigating identity and culture and how the two are intertwined in our personal, familial, and cultural stories becomes the work. Culture shapes identity, but its dominant or received stories are not always one's identity stories. Identity stories, like cultural stories, are contradictory because they are situated, relational, plural, intertextual, fluid, emergent, and co-constitutive (Bava, 2019; Combs & Freedman, 2016). And the racialization of our identities often seeks to be reductionistic, essentialized narratives that are singular and thin, obscuring our intersectionalities and transcontextualized lives. Thus, we need to resist the othering in our clinical engagement by being attuned to how racism operates yet not essentialize our racio-ethnic stories. Instead, be curious how, in everyday interactions, we negotiate and navigate the dynamics of intersecting social locations that Jodie Kliman (2010) identifies as the Social Matrix. Thus, such clinical work requires us to host the complexities with cultural curiosity while allowing the complexity to hold us. Baluran (2023) cautions us against the static construction of race and draws our attention to differential racialization which highlights the dynamism of race and the socio-political processes by which racial categorizations are made and re-made (Zuberi et al., 2015). Such understanding grounds us against binary constructions and essentializing people. We cannot plan our way into these conversations, but we can prepare to host for complexity by becoming curious, noticing relational intersectionality, reflecting on our positionalities, and acting back on the dominant discourse of multiple contexts by honoring client voices and expertise for navigating, negotiating, resisting and/or troubling dominance. Each individual's journey of navigating these complexities is unique, so we cannot pre-determine their path by naming the process for them. Yet, as therapists we can prepare ourselves for what emerges, for each of us, as we stand up to racialization of identities and therapeutic work. And, in the process, in the spaces between our relational and social responsiveness, attuning to the dynamism of cultures and context.

Drawing on discursive practices, I offer dialogic resources to be socio-relationally responsive by hosting the vastness of our contexts and relationships within therapeutic conversations as a way to honor and dignify our client's experiences. To notice how identity-based referential understanding might dupe us into reproducing racism's cultural agenda of essentializing while invisibilizing intersectionality. Instead, to counteract racialization and dominance, I lean into transcontextuality, heterogeneity, the polyphonic stories, and their contradictions by zooming out into the dynamic vastness of our cultural agreements formed and reformed by our socio-relational interactions.

## Reflection Questions

As requested by the editors, I offer these questions in the spirit of informing the conversation for reflection rather than as therapy "tools." These are orienting questions emerging from within the context of the conversation.

### Questions for Therapists

- What is your process, as a therapist, to orient to the relational intersectionality and transcontextuality within the clinical context?
- How do you perform cultural curiosity?
- How do you perform relational and social responsiveness?
- What contradictions, if any, do you see in your identity stories as an Asian American therapist? What forms do these contradictions take (e.g., ethical dilemmas, bodily sensations, silence, tension, etc.)? How do you reclaim these contradictions?

### Questions for Therapy

- How do the concepts of sameness and difference organize your relationship?
- How do you hold contradictions? How do you play with them?
- How are we doing with our conversation in relationship to the consultation you are seeking?
- What else should we be talking about, that we are not talking about? Or how else might we be talking about X [the issue] that would be meaningful for you?

## Notes

1 All client references are case composites to protect client confidentiality. And, the nature of storytelling is that it is partial and limits the fullest sense of play involved

in engaging the complexity. So, these are partial storylines to highlight a specific strand of a much richer interaction.

2   Harris unpacks how race is written into U.S. law as property, which is beyond the scope of this chapter but crucial to understanding the complexity of racism as a while it is simultaneously denied.

3   The terms Asian Americans, U.S.-born Asian, Asian workers in the U.S., transnational Asians, and U.S. Asian population are used interchangeably to refer to adults who self-identify as Asian-origin living in the U.S.

4   The term "project" refers to intentional, organized institutional and systemic efforts over time comprised of many different actors, factors, resources, activities, and assemblages which shape and are shaped by complex, ongoing socio-political processes.

5   Additionally, "the U.S. technology boom of the 1990s and 2000s attracted many high-skilled immigrants, particularly from India and China, to tech centers around the country" (Ruiz, Noe-Bustamante, & Shah, 2023).

6   Though the loop has been described in family therapy textbooks as one of the social justice approaches in family therapy (Gehart, 2023), I offer it here as my journey of sense-making and clinical development rather than a therapy model.

7   To further one's understanding of this process I offer a visualization in the form of a three-min video at: https://www.youtube.com/watch?v=_X4tavN7l-o.

# References

Addison, S., & Coolhart, D. (2015). Expanding the therapy paradigm with queer couples: A relational intersectional lens. *Family Process, 54*(3), 435–453. https://doi.org/10.1111/famp.12171

Andersen, T. (1996). Language is not innocent. In F. Kaslow (Ed.), *The handbook of relational diagnosis* (pp. 119–125). John Wiley & Sons.

Anderson, H. (2012). Collaborative relationships and dialogic conversations: Ideas for a relationally responsive practice. *Family Process, 51*, 8–24. https://doi.org/10.1111/j.1545-5300.2012.01385.x

Anderson, H. (2022). Expressions of the philosophical stance. In H. Anderson & D. Gehart (Eds.), *Collaborative-dialogic practice: Relationships and conversations that make a difference across contexts and cultures* (pp. 19–36). Routledge.

Awad, G. H., Hashem, H., & Nguyen, H. (2021). Identity and ethnic/racial self-labeling among Americans of Arab or Middle Eastern and North African descent. *Identity: An International Journal of Theory and Research, 21*(2), 115–130. https://doi.org/10.1080/15283488.2021.1883277

Badwall, H. (2016). Racialized discourses: Writing against an essentialized story about racism. *Intersectionalities: A Global Journal of Social Work Analysis, Research, Polity, and Practice, 5*(1). https://journals.library.mun.ca/index.php/IJ/article/view/1260

Bakhtin, M. M. (1981). *The dialogic imagination: Four essays.* (C. E. Holquist, Trans.) University of Texas.

Baluran, D. A. (2023). Differential racialization and police interactions among young adults of Asian descent. *Sociology of Race and Ethnicity, 9*(2), 220–234. https://doi.org/10.1177/23326492221125121

Bateson, N. (2023). *Combining.* Triarchy Press.

Bava, S. (2019). Hyperlinked identity: A generative resource in a divisive world. In M. McGoldrick & K. Hardy (Eds.), *Re-visioning family therapy* (pp. 318–335). The Guilford Press.

Bava, S. (2022a). A relationally responsive world: The politics of collaborative-dialogic practices. In H. Anderson & D. Gehart (Eds.), *Collaborative dialogic practice: Relationships and conversations that make a difference across contexts and cultures* (pp. 37–53). Routledge.

Bava, S. (2022b). A guide for conversations: The relational discursive loop. https://medium.com/@thinkplay/a-guide-for-conversations-relational-discursive-loop-6f5ad6a8e3a3

Bava, S., & Greene, M. (2023). *The relational workplace.* ThinkPlay Partners.

Bhatia, S., & Priya, K. R. (2018). Decolonizing culture: Euro-American psychology and the shaping of neoliberal selves in India. *Theory & Psychology, 28*(5), 645–668. https://doi.org/10.1177/0959354318791315

Brown, L. (2009). Cultural competence: A new way of thinking about integration in therapy. *Journal of Psychotherapy Integration, 19*(4), 340–353. https://doi.org/10.1037/a0017967

Coman, S. (2019, August 1). *A brief history of the cultures of Asia.* Retrieved from Smarthistory: https://smarthistory.org/a-brief-history-of-the-cultures-of-asia/

Combs, G., & Freedman, J. (2016). Narrative therapy's relational understanding of identity. *Family Process, 55,* 211–224. https://doi.org/10.1111/famp.12216

Crenshaw, K. (1991). Mapping the margins of intersectionality, identity politics and violence against women of color. *Stanford Law Review, 43,* 1241–1299. https://doi.org/10.2307/1229039

C-SPAN. (2023, April 23). White House Correspondents' Dinner. Retrieved from https://www.c-span.org/video/?527559-1/white-house-correspondents-dinner

Daniels, S. (2022). *The anti-racist organization: Dismantling systemic racism in the workplace.* Wiley.

Falicov, C. (1996). Training to think culturally: A multidimensional comparative framework. *Family Process, 34,* 373–388. https://doi.org/10.1111/j.1545-5300.1995.00373.x.

Fischer, N. L., & Seidman, S. (2016). *Introducing the new sexuality studies.* Taylor & Francis.

Gergen, K. (2023). *An invitation to social construction* (4th ed.). Sage.

Gehart, D. (2023). *Mastering competencies in family therapy: A practical approach to theories and clinical case documentation* (4th ed.). Cengage Learning US.

Gines, K. (2013). Introduction: Critical philosophy of race beyond the black/white binary. *Critical Philosophy of Race, 1*(1), 28–37. https://doi.org/10.5325/critphilrace.1.1.0028

Hardy, B., & Ness, O. (2015). Beyond the therapeutic state. *European Journal of Psychotherapy & Counselling, 17*(4), 322–325. https://doi.org/10.1080/13642537.2015.1096813

Harpalani, V. (2013). DesiCrit: Theorizing the racial ambiguity of south Asian Americans. *69 NYU Annual Survey of American Law 77 Chicago-Kent College of Law Research Paper No. 2013-30, 69,* pp. 77–184. Retrieved from https://papers.ssrn.com/sol3/papers.cfm?abstract_id=2308892

Harris, C. (2020). Reflections on whiteness as property. *Harvard Law Review, 134*(1), 1–10.

Klein, E., & Mills, C. (2017). Psy-Expertise, therapeutic culture and the politics of the personal in development. *Third World Quarterly, 38*(9), 1990–2008. https://doi.org /10.1080/01436597.2017.1319277

Kliman, J. (2010). Intersections of social privilege and marginalization: A visual teaching tool. In J. Ariel, P. Hernández-Wolfe, & S. Stearns, *AFTA Monograph Series: Expanding our social justice practices: Advances in theory and training* (pp. 39–48). American Family Therapy Academy.

Kohn, M., & Reddy, K. (2023). "Colonialism". In Edward N. Zalta & Uri Nodelman (Eds.), *The Stanford encyclopedia of philosophy* (Spring 2023 ed.). Retrieved November 15, 2023, from https://plato.stanford.edu/archives/spr2023/entries/colonialism/

Lee, J., & Ramakrishnan, K. (2020). Who counts as Asian. *Ethnic and Racial Studies, 43*(10), 1733–1756. https://doi.org/10.1080/01419870.2019.1671600

Lee, J., & Zhou, M. (2015). *The Asian American achievement paradox.* Russell Sage Foundation.

Lorde, A. (2020). *Sister outsider.* Penguin.

McDonough, M. (2022). This lovely thing we do together: Collaborative-dialogic practice through a literary lens. In H. Anderson, & D. Gehart (Eds.), *Collaborative-Dialogic practice* (pp. 69-81). Routledge.

McDowell, T., Knudson-Martin, C., & Bermudez, M. J. (2022). *Socioculturally attuned family therapy* (2nd ed.). Taylor & Francis.

McNamee, S. (2008). Transformative dialogue: Coordinating conflicting moralities. *The Lindberg Lecture 2008.* Retrieved July 17, 2022. https://mypages.unh.edu/sheilamc-namee/publications/transformative-dialogue-coordinating-conflicting-moralities

Menakem, R. (2017). *My grandmother's hands.* Central Recovery Press.

Mignolo, W. D. (2021). *The politics of decolonial investigations.* Duke University Press.

Purdie-Vaughns, V., & Eibach, R. P. (2008). Intersectional invisibility: The distinctive advantages and disadvantages of multiple subordinate-group identities. *Sex Roles, 59,* 377–391. https://doi.org/10.1007/s11199-008-9424-4

Ruiz, N. G., Noe-Bustamante, L., & Shah, S. (2023, May 8). *Diverse cultures and shared experiences shape Asian American identities.* Retrieved from Pew Research Center: https://www.pewresearch.org/race-ethnicity/2023/05/08/diverse-cultures-and-shared -experiences-shape-asian-american-identities/#fnref-1665-1

Sheinberg, M., & Fraenkel, P. (2000). *The relational trauma of incest: A family-based approach to treatment.* Guilford Publications.

Shotter, J. (2015a). On being dialogical: An ethics of attunement. *Context,* 137, 8–11 .

Shotter, J. (2015b). Tom Andersen, fleeting events, the bodily feelings they arouse in us, and the dialogical: Transitory understandings and action guiding anticipations. *Australian and New Zealand Journal of Family Therapy, 36,* 72–87. https://doi.org /10.1002/anzf.1087

Shotter, J. (2016). *Speaking, actually: Towards a new "fluid" common-sense understanding of relational becomings.* Everything Connected Press.

Sue, S., Sue, D., & Sue, D. W. (2021). Who are the Asian Americans? Commentary on the Asian American psychology special issue. *American Psychologist, 76*(4), 689–692. https://doi.org/10.1037/amp0000825

Sugarman, J. (2015). Neoliberalism and psychological ethics. *Journal of Theoretical and Philosophical Psychology, 35*(2), 103–116. https://apa.org/pubs/journals/features/teo -a0038960.pdf

Sullum, J. (2020, July). Curing the therapeutic state: Thomas Szasz interviewed by Jacob Sullum. *Reason*, p. 28 ''et seq.''. http://reason.com/archives/2000/07/01/curing-the -therapeutic-state-t

TimeMaps. (n.d.). *European World Empires*. Retrieved from TimeMap: https://timemaps .com/civilizations/european-world-empires/

Westmoreland, P. (2013). Racism in a Black White binary_ on the reaction to Trayvon Martin. https://scholarship.law.ufl.edu/csrrr_events/10thspringlecture/panels/7/

Yancy, G., & Kim, D. H. (2015, October 8). *The Invisible Asian. The New York Times*. https://archive.nytimes.com/opinionator.blogs.nytimes.com/2015/10/08/the-invisible -asian/

Yip, T., Cheah, C. S., Kiang, L., & Hall, G. C. (2021). Rendered invisible: Are Asian Americans a model or a marginalized minority? *American Psychologist, 76*(4), 575– 581. https://doi.org/10.1037/amp0000857

Zhou, L. (2021, May 5). *The inadequacy of the term "Asian American."* Vox. https:// www.vox.com/identities/22380197/asian-american-pacific-islander-aapi-heritage -anti-asian-hate-attacks

Zuberi, T., Patterson, E. J., & Stewart, Q. T. (2015). Race, methodology, and social construction in the genomic era. *Annals AAPSS, 661*, 109–127. https://doi.org/10.1177 /0002716215589718

# Chapter 2

# Unraveling Asian American Stereotypes

The Model Minority Myth, Honorary Whiteness, and Forever Foreigner

*Hoa N. Nguyen*

> *because our ancestors knew solidarity even if they couldn't pronounce it. They made a sound. We make a sound. Our chants, and screams, and drums, and cries will chase after all the miles you've tried to run from us. We are not quiet. We are not submissive. We have always been fighters.*
>
> (Excerpt from "Asian American History" by Khoi the Poet 2016)

As Asian Americans are weaving our own stories about who we are and what our experiences are like in a white-dominant culture, stereotypes such as the model minority myth, honorary white, and perpetual or forever foreigner (Tuan, 1998) tell a single narrative about the Asian American experience. At best, they are narrow and presumptive, couched in preconceived generalizations and monolithic representations of an expansive, diverse group of people. At worst, they conceal the oppressive and dehumanizing experiences Asian people experience in the United States. This chapter will discuss the history and ongoing racialization of stereotypes about Asian American experiences and explore clinical considerations for broadening and transcending these assumptions.

## Model Minority Myth: Obscuring the Complexities and Inequities in the Lives of Asian Americans

> *Asian Americans inhabit a purgatorial status: neither white enough nor black enough, unmentioned in most conversations about racial identity. In the popular imagination, Asian Americans are all high-achieving professionals. But in reality, this is the most economically divided group in the country, a tenuous alliance of people with roots from South Asia to East Asia to the Pacific Islands, from tech millionaires to service industry laborers. How do we speak honestly about the Asian American condition—if such a thing exists?*
>
> (Hong, 2020)

DOI: 10.4324/9781003321590-4

The model minority myth is a longstanding stereotype that obscures complexities and fails to portray the breadth and depth of diversity within the experiences of Asian people in the United States (Walton & Truong, 2023). Although the term was not referenced directly, the idea of the model minority was introduced by white American sociologist William Petersen in 1966 in a *New York Times* article (Petersen, 1966; Shih et al., 2019), in which Japanese Americans were propped as examples of "successful minorities." It is critical to note the contextual backdrop that existed when the model minority stereotype was created—the sociopolitical context of the 1950s–1960s, the tensions between Black and white America, and the struggle for justice and equality during the civil rights movement. The origins of the model minority myth further highlight how it has been used as a tool of whiteness to maintain dominant racial ideologies, establish racial hierarchies, delegitimize the rights and freedoms of African Americans, and deny Asian Americans' experiences of racism and oppression.

### The Model Minority Myth as a Racial Wedge

A key criticism of the model minority myth is the comparison of Asian Americans to other racially minoritized groups, proposing people of Asian descent are able to overcome the barriers of racial and structural discrimination (Whaley & Noel, 2013). In this vein, the model minority myth has been manufactured to effectively draw a divide between Asian Americans and other racial minorities (e.g., African Americans, Latino Americans, etc.) by juxtaposing the successes of one racial minority against others. Further, the stereotype emphasizes how individual strength, morality, hard work, and grit are all that are necessary for any racial minority to overcome systemic racism. These stereotypes do nothing to serve Asian Americans and other racial minorities. Being rewarded as the "good" minority reifies conformity to dominant whiteness. Being white is established as the top of the racial hierarchy in which everyone must reach. Studies have explored the impact of internalizing the model minority myth. For instance, Asian American students demonstrate an awareness of a "racial hierarchy" with whiteness as both the measurement and the top of the hierarchy (Park, 2011). Going beyond the metric of whiteness is necessary to gain a fuller understanding of Asian American experiences (Xu & Lee, 2013; Wing, 2007).

### Internalizing the Model Minority Myth

Trieu and Lee (2018) explain how "it is within this oppressive colonial structure that the colonial subjects can potentially begin to believe, internalize, and project the shame of who they are" (p. 68). Families who internalize the model minority stereotype may find pride in and profess the myth to be true, but their internalization of such stereotypes does not exist within a vacuum. In spite of the racism, there is a societal desire to be accepted, recognized, and to thrive in

Western society. One example is Chua's (2012) book *Battle Hymn of the Tiger Mother*, a controversial book that discusses the role of parenting practices and values in the educational success of Asian Americans. While the memoir may be reflective of Chua's personal experiences, it has been criticized for emphasizing the model minority myth and crystallizing the stereotype of Asian parents as strict, authoritarian, and stoic (Shih et al., 2019). As a minority race, some Asian families may be drawn to identifying with a sense of cultural excellence as a way to cope with the minority stressors or to take advantage of the perceived benefits of being seen as the "best minority" and conform to Western society. In reality, this false sense of racial superiority only serves to add pressure to assimilate and adhere to American racialized ideals (Subramanian, 2019).

When parents internalize the model minority myth, it can lead to elevated levels of stress, anxiety, and skewed expectations for children and adolescents (Rodriguez-Operana, 2017; Yim, 2009). Asian parents and children who internalize this stereotype may also feel dissonance or displaced self-blame when they encounter the realities of racial discrimination but misinterpret their experience as some fault of their own. When encountering overt discrimination, they may interpret oppressive experiences as their own failure and shortcomings, resulting in self-doubt and shame instead of being able to identify the sources of racism and cultural discrimination. The pressure to live up to the model minority myth and deny one's own experiences of racism and discrimination creates immense pressure to succeed and has been attributed to the high suicide rates and low mental health service utilization in the Asian American community (Noh, 2018). This is consistent with research that demonstrates how internalized racism of positive Asian American stereotypes discourages help-seeking behavior and correlates with higher psychological distress (Gupta et al., 2011). Ultimately, internalizing the model minority stereotype is in essence internalizing the oppressive narratives that invalidate the experiences of Asian Americans (Hwang, 2021).

### Not All Asians Look (or Achieve) the Same

The model minority myth creates a monolithic image of perceived success among all Asian ethnic groups. It is often that the behaviors and actions—both failures and successes—of individuals from a racial minority group are attributed to the entire cultural group, whereas the actions of individuals from a majority racial group are defined on the basis of individual motivations, ability, and circumstances. This demonstrates the insidious nature of telling a single narrative about minority racial groups. Contrary to being a monolith, Asian Americans are the largest group of immigrants since 2010 and the fastest-growing with an increase of 81% from 2000 to 2019 (Budiman & Ruiz, 2021). Categorized under one racial, ethnic umbrella, they trace their heritage across expansive cultural, linguistic, ethnic, migration, and socioeconomic differences (Yip et al., 2021).

The model minority myth is a double-edged sword. In placing Asian Americans on a pedestal, the stereotype robs us of our individuality and reinforces the idea that racism is no longer a problem (Shih et al., 2019). By homogenizing Asian American experiences, we assume people of Asian descent do not experience racially-based social disadvantages (Liu-Countryman, 2017; Lee et al., 2017). In actuality, income and education are considerably different among Asian Americans, as the most economically fractioned racial and ethnic group (Kochhar & Cilluffo, 2018). Some Asian ethnic groups have consistently reported some of the lowest unemployment rates and longest duration of unemployment (Ramakrishnan & Ahmad, 2014). Regardless of one's credentials or skill set, Asian Americans are least likely among all racial groups to be promoted to management roles (Gee & Peck, 2018). There is also stark contrast in income, wealth, home ownership, and education between those who immigrated with higher educational attainment and refugees who immigrated with limited access to education (Shih et al., 2019). The misconception that Asian Americans have, as a whole, achieved economically and financially, masks the great disparity, poverty, and income inequality Asians face (Yip et al., 2021).

## Honorary Whiteness: Understanding the Colonial Roots and Fantasy of Being White-Adjacent

*When I hear the phrase 'Asians are next in line to be white,' I replace the word 'white' with 'disappear.' Asians are next in line to disappear.*

(Hong, 2021)

In internalizing the model minority myth, Asian identities and experiences are veiled by stereotypes that perceive Asian Americans as white-adjacent. The honorary white label assumes Asian Americans are given access to privileges and social advantages, similar to or on par with white Americans (Lee, 2020). Historically, the term "honorary white" originated from South Africa's apartheid legislation of the 1950s which divided the country's population into race-based binaries of either European (white) or non-European, racially segregating, denying educational and occupational rights to people of color and prohibiting racial intermingling (Park, 2008). As a political term, "honorary white" was a political status that granted some rights and privileges to Japanese people, while continually classifying them as non-white and excluding other Asian ethnic groups such as the local Chinese people. Less attention has been paid to the anti-apartheid movements in Asia that rejected honorary whiteness, protested against apartheid, and called for global solidarity (Makino, 2016). As an ideological tool of colonialism that maintains white supremacy, honorary whiteness is yet another way to establish and maintain racial hierarchies (Sibango, 2022).

Anthropologist Ong (2006) refers to "honorary whiteness" as a fantasy in which the individual receives privileges contingent on them defining themselves based on the colonizer-self. This process of identifying with and conforming to the colonizer-self inevitably denies parts of ourselves. To retain the honorary white status, we have to repress or reject parts of ourselves to fit the mold. We also have to reject and exclude other racial groups or even members within our own racial group that do not meet the white standard. Falling into the honorary white trope is alluring in its promise for heightened status in Western society. However, this status is conditional and relies on continued conformity to the colonial system that maintains white supremacy (Young, 2009). The fantasy of honorary whiteness is rooted in awarding power and legitimacy to white, eurocentric Western ways of thinking, behaving, and being. This further highlights the sense of racial, ethnic isolation, and invisibility associated with the perceptions of Asian Americans as white- or privilege-adjacent (Clemons, 2019; Yi Borromeo, 2018).

In addition, the illusive honorary white label fades when taking into account the continued and increasing incidents of anti-Asian hate crimes and racism (Wang et al., 2021; Wu & Nguyen, 2022). Being perceived as white-adjacent does not prohibit anti-Asian racism and discrimination or protect one from it. Elevated levels of anti-Asian racism are found to negatively influence Asian American mental health (Louie-Poon et al., 2022). Asian immigrants and Asian Americans reported higher levels of mental disorders than white Americans during the COVID-19 pandemic, linked to their experiences of stigmatization, violence, and racial discrimination (Wu et al., 2021). During the pandemic, Asian Americans reported experiencing COVID-related stress and fear of racism and discrimination (Huang & Tsai, 2023; Huynh et al., 2022). It is no surprise anti-Asian racism has a direct impact on the mental and physical health of Asian and Asian Americans, showing how the honorary white status is always tentative and provisional.

I remember watching a video clip of a KKK rally against Vietnamese fishers in the 1980s, in which Vietnamese fishers were targeted and harassed for entering the fishing industry in Texas, Louisiana, and other coastal states. It was a history I had not learned or delved into as deeply before. I was raised in Atlanta, Georgia, where I was fortunate enough to have been exposed to critical perspectives on American history of racism and colonialism. However, exploring the narratives of Asian Americans beyond the black-white chasm was a newer realization that challenged the model minority myth and honorary whiteness. As an Asian American, I was not exposed to the ways we were and have long been a part of America's history of racism. I lived mostly with the guise that "it was not that bad for us" which both normalized anti-Asian sentiments and obscured the discrimination Asian Americans faced. Seeing the video helped me see how we were deeply a part of the fabric of this history, both as pawns against other racial minorities and as victims/survivors of white supremacy.

## Forever Foreigner Fallacy: But Where Are You Really From?

*As a professor and licensed therapist in South Georgia, I am encased in a bubble of educational privilege within the University setting, but when*

*I step into the local community, I am often reminded of the way I am perceived by others. I often tell my students the story of a casual conversation with a local community member in which I am asked "Are you a dreamer?" Naively, I answered, "Sure! I'm a dreamer. I have dreams and goals for the future" to which the person responded, "No, I mean the illegal kind."*

Being perceived as a DACA (Deferred Action for Childhood Arrivals) recipient is not so much a personal offense as it was a stark reminder of how Asian Americans are still perceived in our culture and society. The foreigner fallacy stems from Orientalism, a colonial, Eurocentric notion that frames the "Orient" as exotic, inferior, and threatening to Western society (Said, 2003). Orientalism is also a form of "othering" in which one group forms a dichotomous view of us versus them that often leads to marginalizing and excluding other groups they perceive as different or "other" (Banerjee et al., 2020). In othering Asian people, society objectifies and dehumanizes, reducing us to an assumed or perceived Asian aesthetic and phenotype, despite the vast diversity in the facial and phenotypic characteristics across all Asian groups. As long as society exoticizes and homogenizes Asians and Asian Americans, it will continue to perceive us as other, foreign, and un-American.

### Asian American History Is American History

Asian Americans continue to be viewed as the perpetual foreigner, despite history documenting long-standing Chinese immigration that dates back to the 19th century (Lee, 2015). At that time, Chinese workers were blamed for stealing jobs from white American laborers. This is indicative of the "yellow peril" notion which fueled societal fear, racism, and xenophobic sentiments against Chinese immigrants (see Chapter 5). Chinese immigrants continued to endure racial discrimination and violence into the 20th century, along with different Asian groups that arrived such as Korean, Japanese, Hindu, and Filipino immigrants (Sabharwal et al., 2022). The Asian American community has encountered acts of racism and violence throughout American history, including but not limited to the Chinese Exclusion Act of 1882; the Chinese massacre of 1871, one of the worst mass lynchings of an immigrant group; the forced internment of Japanese Americans during World War II; discriminatory housing, education, land ownership, and citizenship rights practices against Korean immigrants in the 1900s; stereotypes and similar barriers to rights for South Asian immigrants; the KKK attacks on Southeast Asians post Vietnam War; the murder of Vincent Chin and other similar cases; racial discrimination and attacks targeting South Asians based on their skin color and due to anti-Muslim prejudice post 9/11; and the Atlanta spa shootings driven by the intersection of racialized exoticism and hypersexualization that took the lives of six women of Asian descent (Lee, 2015; Mineo, 2021).

While the view of Asian Americans as more foreign and less American has lessened from 2007 to 2020, this implicit bias grew after the use of stigmatizing language in the media that attributed blame to China for the COVID-19 pandemic (Daley et al., 2022; Darling-Hammond, 2020). Recent surges in anti-Asian violence have been linked to the perception of COVID-19 as the "Kung Flu" or "Chinese virus" and the scapegoating of Asian Americans during a public health emergency. Asian and Asian Americans reported instances of COVID-19-related discrimination at two times higher rates than white Americans (Wu et al., 2021). Stereotypes about racial minorities tend to bolster in economic slumps (Bianchi et al., 2018) and in relation to increases in minority populations (Zou & Cheryan, 2022). Kang (2022) argues that the forever foreigner stereotype will pervade until Asian American history is included in K-12 education. When there is increased societal consciousness of how Asian Americans have been part of the fabric of U.S. history and rooted in the construction of America and its constitution, it may be more difficult for these biases to fluctuate based on sociopolitical and economic changes.

### The Paradox and Dialectics of Asian Stereotypes

Paradoxically, the forever foreigner stereotype counters the model minority myth and honorary white stereotype. While the model minority myth and honorary white label serves as ways to distinguish Asian Americans in the measure of racial superiority maintained by white-dominant culture, it is also quickly diminished by negative portrayals of Asian immigrants as a social and economic threat (Mudambi, 2019). The paradox of being perceived as a perpetual foreigner has been linked to experiences of internalizing psychological distress for Asian American youth (Park et al., 2021) and burnout for Asian Americans in the local government and the public sector (Le & Barboza-Wilkes, 2022). These stereotypes establish two contradictory narratives, one in which Asian people are viewed to be so alien to the U.S. culture that they have not assimilated at all, and one in which they have assimilated so well, they might as well be white (Zhou, 2012). As two sides of the same coin, they both serve to legitimize the marginalization of Asians as an invisible minority. Interestingly, in one study, while Asian Americans are perceived as less American than white Americans, they report feeling no less American than other racial groups and are conscious of how they are perceived by others (Cheryan & Monin, 2005). In addition, Asian Americans in the study did not distance themselves from their Asian identity, despite being denied their American identity. Cheryan and Monin propose the possibility that Asian Americans did not feel one identity negated the other, and "it was possible to be both 100% Asian and 100% American" (2005, p. 726).

## Personal Connection to the Topic

As a 1.5-generation Vietnamese who immigrated with her family via a government-sponsored refugee program when I was five years old, I grew up with very limited representations of Asian Americans that did not resonate with my own experience. When I was younger, I never thought of myself as Asian. The term "Asian American" had been an arbitrary label given to me from a Western, U.S.-centric lens. The U.S. media was littered with Asian American stereotypes, including ones that either painted Asian women as docile and submissive or as hypersexualized dragon ladies. This did not represent any of the Asian women I knew, but they reflected the way some people viewed us and the narratives that had been ascribed to Asian women from a white-dominant lens. As a child in the United States, I also remember being told by an older white American man to watch *Miss Saigon*, a Broadway debut in 1989 that tells the story of a romance between a U.S. soldier and a Vietnamese woman during the Vietnam War. He regarded the performance as a seminal insight into the history of the Vietnam War and, therefore, critical for me to view as a Vietnamese person. Watching Miss Saigon brings forth mixed feelings for me. Did I love how beautiful and talented the actress, Lea Salonga, was as the main protagonist? Yes. Was I uneased by the negative portrayals of Vietnamese people? Also, yes.

When there are more diverse examples, the occasional imperfect attempt at representation may be more forgivable. However, since Asian American representation is so few and far in between, especially during those times, these portrayals can hold weight in our everyday interactions and relationships. For instance, the family member of a boyfriend I once dated admitted she felt very protective of him and wanted to make sure I wasn't "dating him just for his money like the prostitute character in *Miss Saigon*." Despite having exposure to other Asian people before, the image of *Miss Saigon* was still imprinted in the person's bias, showing how impactful stereotypes can be. The musical has been critiqued for being imbued with every racist, orientalist trope possible, from the negative representations of Viet men as money-hungry to the characterization of Viet women as sex workers. The storyline centers on a white savior fantasy by portraying Vietnamese people as inferior to white Americans and as solely victims, devoid of agency (Jung, 2021).

### Remembering My Family

This was not the story I saw or heard in my family and community. The stories I witnessed were ones of courage and endurance, loss and regeneration, and a deep remembrance of their cultural roots and ancestry. My brother-in-law fled the Vietnam war at 17 years old by boat without his parents and lived in a refugee camp in Malaysia before being transferred to the Philippines and then to the United States. My sisters navigated the complexities of living in two cultural worlds as third culture kids. They were teased at school for wearing their cheongsam-style tops, before cheongsams/qipaos were popularized as oriental or jacquard dresses in Western brands Zara and Urban Outfitters or featured in high fashion design such as Louis Vuitton, Gucci, and Dolce & Gabbana. My father survived as a prisoner of war for seven years before bringing his family to the United States. My mother started her own alteration shop where she worked as a seasoned seamstress with more than 30 years of experience. After surviving the Vietnam War, my family started their life in a new land and country, adjusting to a different language, community, and culture.

The generational stories of survival in my family counters these one-dimensional Asian American stereotypes. Our strength and resilience emanates from our culturally rooted experiences and legacies, not from a measure of closeness to whiteness. While my family was more fortunate than others, I know of other members in my Vietnamese community who still struggle with poverty and lack of access to resources. For us, this culminated in a sense of gratitude and a recognition that while our circumstances have drastically improved, many members of our community are still working through economic disparities and disadvantages. We have fought against the narratives of honorary white and model minority myth. At the same time, we have had to externalize narratives of white superiority. I remember learning as a child about French colonization of Vietnam, in which members of the older generation in my family stated, "The French civilized us." This statement was vexing and infuriating, but indicative of the strong hold that colonization has on our sense of cultural identity, self-worth, and value. I know of aunties who considered marrying a white person as either equally attractive or even more attractive than marrying a member of our own race, internalizing the dominant narratives of whiteness as better. We have to actively challenge and understand how we absorb these assumptions, by reflecting on, connecting to, and learning about our personal, family, and cultural histories, especially the generational wisdom that helped facilitate our survival.

## Clinical Case Example

Linh Nguyen is a 28-year-old Asian American woman of Vietnamese descent, who immigrated to the United States with her family at the age of 10, and was raised in a white-majority suburban community. She grew up having dealt with racial slurs and being ostracized for her perceived cultural and linguistic differences. To survive the school environment as a child, she became adept at navigating two cultural worlds—the Asian household she grew up in and larger white-dominant culture. Her mother's recent death has her grappling with uncertainties around how to honor her mother's legacy and navigate conflicts regarding traditional Vietnamese mourning practices. Her grief and pain is layered with questioning her sense of identity as she feels ashamed of never having learned more about Vietnamese heritage and practices from her mother while she was alive.

The therapist begins therapy by unpacking her family history and the cultural dynamics around grief and mourning for Linh. As she shares the emotional aspects of the loss of her mom, she shares having lost a close and supportive relationship and also one of her few connections to the family's cultural legacy. She admitted not knowing much about her mother's upbringing or history as they never dove deeply into the family history. When asked by the therapist what was the foundation for their closeness, Linh reflected on how her mother always showed her love through actions such as preparing her food. Now that her mother had passed, she wished she had spent more time cooking with her mom and learning different Vietnamese dishes from her.

### Subverting Racialized Stereotypes

While processing her emotions and grief, the therapist explores how Linh's Vietnamese heritage and the American culture in which she was raised inform the cultural rituals she wishes to include in honoring her mom: "What parts of both cultures do you want to include?" Linh responds, acknowledging how a large part of Vietnamese culture is setting an altar in their homes to venerate their ancestors, but also showed some hesitation, stating that her white friend regarded altars as unhealthy coping, stating, "It sounds like you don't let go of the dead if you have an altar for them." Linh was taken aback by hearing this preconceived bias against a mourning practice in her culture. She wondered for a moment if it was healthy or not.

The friend continued, "But you're basically white—I mean American—so it's not like the altar is something you're into, right?" Again, Linh paused as she felt mixed feelings, both irritated and uncertain about what her friend said. The therapist began to explore the meaning and assumptions behind these statements and how they affected Linh. Linh was able to explore how the friend unknowingly made disparaging assumptions about her Vietnamese mourning practices, only to follow it up with the suggestion that she was more white-adjacent and not really "Vietnamese" anyways.

The therapist mindfully unpacked how mourning looked different in Vietnamese and American culture, and varied ways people in every culture grieved differently to acknowledge both inter- and intra-group differences.

> It seems honoring one's loved one in a home altar allows the person to continue a relationship and connection with their family member, which is found in grief research to be a critical component of being able to grieve and mourn in meaningful ways.

The therapist then asked Linh what she believes her mom would have wanted, and also how she feels having her mom's altar in the home would continue their closeness. Linh responded that if her mom's altar is in the home, she would be able to cook for her mom and prepare her meals during her death anniversary as a yearly ritual. The therapist reflected how this seemed like a way for them to "cook together" and for her to continue to learn her mom's dishes and share the cultural legacy with her mom in this way. While Linh conducted much of the funeral ceremony at an American venue with some integrated Vietnamese American traditions, she was able to set up the altar in a way that represented her connection to her mom and her heritage.

### Shame and Bicultural Identity

As Linh subverted the negative stereotypes of Asian heritage in relation to mourning and grief, she discovered a sense of shame around not being Vietnamese enough, which surfaced when she explored some of the Vietnamese traditions around extended family that seem unfamiliar to her. She felt a pressure to have a stronger connection to her heritage. Friends of the family sometimes commented on how "Americanized" she is and took note of moments when she spoke the language with an American accent. At the same time, she also felt invisible when she was in conversations with friends who showed a lack of understanding or curiosity about her cultural differences. In another instance, she expressed annoyance when a friend sent her a request for a Thai recipe, assuming she would know how to cook Thai food. This was not uncommon in Linh's experience, making her feel more invisible when friends group her into a broad Asian category. There was a sense of shame when she encountered friends who had not regarded her as Vietnamese at all, and in this aspect, she felt more invisible and unseen.

One of the goals of therapy is Linh rediscovering her relationship with her mother in her loss and keeping that part alive in honor of her mom. Another goal is rediscovering her relationship with herself, her identity, and cultural identity. For her, as for many, losing a mother can be a life-changing event that shifts a person's sense of identity. This uncertain place could become new grounds for Linh to learn more about herself, her mom, and her family culture. The therapist helped reframe these uncertainties around the funeral ceremony as opportunities to ask questions and talk to family members to get to know her mom through the lens of others. In these family interviews, driven by her curiosity about her mom, Linh found stories of pride, hardship, and resilience in her mother's dangerous journey as one of the Vietnamese boat people. She pieced together parts of the history she learned from different family members and researched reading materials such as *The Vietnamese Boat People* by Nguy Vu and David Maruyama to better understand her family's history.

### Inclusion and Belonging: Embracing Liminality

Only by embracing the liminal spaces between her not being quite American and not quite Vietnamese can Linh integrate both and see how being Vietnamese does not counter her being American, and vice versa. The therapist helped facilitate this idea with a conversation on the liminality of food, and how staple Vietnamese foods (phở, bánh mì, bánh xèo) were all influenced by French colonists, and now, in turn, Vietnamese food is gaining popularity and influencing American culture. Had one not known the origin of these foods, they would merely be accepted and digested as part of the culture. Because of the significance of food in Linh's relationship with her mother, it served as a powerful metaphor for liminality and inclusion. As such, it offered a useful starting point to discuss how fusing different cultures does make the dish half Vietnamese, half French, but rather it has transformed into a third entity altogether.

As Bateson (1972) proposed the whole is greater than the sum of its parts, understanding cultural identity experiences for Asian Americans exists in the same vein, in which not one part or culture in separation can define the person. A person's cultural identity has to be understood within all its interconnections. To thicken this narrative with more in-depth examples, the therapist recommended Linh dive into other complex stories of the Asian American experience, such as *The Farewell*, a film exploring grief from a Chinese American lens, *Crying in H Mart*, the memoir of a Korean American who lost her mother to cancer and found solace and cultural connection through food, and *Family Style: Memoirs of an American from Vietnam*, a graphic memoir on a Vietnamese immigrant's journey for belonging. Linh is encouraged to tell her own story, one rooted in the cultural complexities of who she is and who she is becoming.

### Shedding the Model Minority Myth, Forever Foreigner, and Other Invisibility Cloaks

> *If the Asian American consciousness must be emancipated, we must free ourselves of our conditional existence.*
>
> (Hong, 2021, p. 202)

Asian Americans exist based on the conditions of white-dominant culture and supremacy in which belonging is a promise just out of reach (Hong, 2021), and the stereotypes of model minority, forever foreigner, and honorary white are invisibility cloaks that erase the complexity and intersectionality of our stories. They reinforce harmful stereotypes, lead to feelings of alienation, and oversimplify the systemic inequalities within the broad, diverse group of Asian Americans. By shedding these cloaks, we can strive for a more equitable society that values the multifaceted experiences of racial minorities and recognizes the rich diversity of our members. While being visible is a critical step, we also need to be willing to ask for more depth and complexity in the ways Asian immigrants and Asian Americans are represented and perceived. Increased visibility at times can correlate with the increase in violence, as the rise of anti-Asian hate crimes occurred despite growing Asian American representation in Hollywood, social media, and pop culture (Luna, n.d.).

The process of shedding these stereotypes can include but is not limited to:

- learning about the history and present-day struggles, concerns, and experiences of Asian Americans;
- highlighting the stories of resilience, strengths, and movers and shakers that resisted and confronted anti-Asian racism;
- addressing issues of shame and mental health stigma;
- pushing for more visibility in the workplace, cinema, government, policy, and other public arenas of society;
- celebrating the richness and diversity of Asian cultural heritages, values, and traditions;
- engaging the intergenerational wisdom across Asian families and communities; and
- crafting our own individual and collective stories with attention to complexity, depth, intersectionality, and humanity.

The impact of rejecting societally imposed identities is cultivating the freedom to be truly seen and perhaps even more importantly to truly see ourselves. It also allows us to break stereotypes and liberates us to be both an individual and part of a diverse, collective cultural group. Finally, it combats Asian caricatures and stereotypes that rob us of our humanity by re-humanizing us.

## Reflection Questions

### Questions for the Therapist

- How have you experienced or observed the perpetuation of racialized stereotypes, such as the myth of model minority, forever foreigner, or honorary white in your professional and/or personal life?
- What assumptions have you or other colleagues made about Asian families? How do you counter these problematic assumptions about Asian Americans?
- What would it be like for Asian Americans to tell stories about themselves, their families, and their lives from a perspective, in a manner that is rooted in their own cultural experiences rather than stereotypes?
- How do you challenge narratives of shame in bi-/multicultural experiences as a therapist?
- What complexities are embodied in today's Asian American family experiences?
- In what ways can Asian American therapists find their therapeutic voice amid white dominant culture of therapy?'

## Questions for Therapy

- In what ways do people (those around you and society as whole) misunderstand or misrepresent your racial identity? What assumptions have they made?
- How does it feel to be grouped as an Asian American?
- What are times in which you feel most seen, heard, or understood in your racial identity? How do you experience this?
- What would it mean for you to own and embrace your experiences? What parts of your racial experience are you most proud of?
- Who can you share these stories with? How does their understanding of your racial identity impact how you see/understand yourself?

# References

Banerjee, D., Kallivayalil, R. A., & Rao, T. S. (2020). The 'othering' in pandemics: Prejudice and orientalism in COVID-19. *Indian Journal of Social Psychiatry, 36*(Suppl 1), S102–S106. https://doi.org/10.4103/ijsp.ijsp_261_20

Bateson, G. (1972). *Steps to an ecology of mind.* Jason Aronson.

Bianchi, E. C., Hall, E. V., & Lee, S. (2018). Reexamining the link between economic downturns and racial antipathy: Evidence that prejudice against blacks rises during recessions. *Psychological Science, 29*(10), 1584–1597. https://doi.org/10.1177/0956797618777214

Budiman, A., & Ruiz, N. G. (2021). *Asian Americans are the fastest-growing racial or ethnic group in the US.* www.pewresearch.org/short-reads/2021/04/09/asian-americans-are-the-fastest-growing-racial-or-ethnic-group-in-the-u-s/

Cheryan, S., & Monin, B. (2005). Where are you really from?: Asian Americans and identity denial. *Journal of Personality and Social Psychology, 89*(5), 717–730. https://doi.org/10.1037/0022-3514.89.5.717

Chua, A. (2012). *Battle hymn of the tiger mother.* Bloomsbury Publishing PLC.

Clemons, C. L. (2019). *Model minority expectations: Exploring with young Chinese American college students who seek career counselling.* [Doctoral dissertation] Fordham University.

Daley, J. S., Gallagher, N. M., & Bodenhausen, G. V. (2022). The pandemic and the "perpetual foreigner": How threats posed by the COVID-19 pandemic relate to stereotyping of Asian Americans. *Frontiers in Psychology, 13*, 821–891. https://doi.org/10.3389/fpsyg.2022.821891

Darling-Hammond, S., Michaels, E. K., Allen, A. M., Chae, D. H., Thomas, M. D., Nguyen, T. T., Mahasin, M. M., & Johnson, R. C. (2020). After "the China virus" went viral: Racially charged coronavirus coverage and trends in bias against Asian Americans. *Health Education & Behavior, 47*(6), 870–879. https://doi.org/10.1177/10901981209579

Gee, B., & Peck, D. (2018). Metrics of the glass ceiling at the intersection of race and gender. *Strategic HR Review, 17*(3), 110–118. https://doi.org/10.1108/SHR-03-2018-0023

Gupta, A., Szymanski, D. M., & Leong, F. T. (2011). The "model minority myth": Internalized racialism of positive stereotypes as correlates of psychological distress, and attitudes toward help-seeking. *Asian American Journal of Psychology, 2*(2), 101–114. https://doi.org/10.1037/a0024183

Hong, C. P. (2020). *Minor feelings: An Asian American reckoning.* One World.

Huang, C. Y., & Tsai, W. (2023). Asian American parents' experiences of stress, discrimination, and mental health during COVID-19. *Families, Systems, & Health, 41*(1), 68–77. https://doi.org/10.1037/fsh0000715

Huynh, V. W., Raval, V. V., & Freeman, M. (2022). Ethnic-racial discrimination towards Asian Americans amidst COVID-19, the so-called "China" virus and associations with mental health. *Asian American Journal of Psychology, 13*(3), 259–269. https://doi.org/10.1037/aap0000264

Hwang, W. C. (2021). Demystifying and addressing internalized racism and oppression among Asian Americans. *American Psychologist, 76*(4), 596. https://doi.org/10.1037/amp0000798

Jung, S. (2021). Miss Saigon: The Asian experience in the perspective of the white man. *Asian American Research Journal, 1*(1), 1–8. https://doi.org/10.5070/RJ41153720

Kang, L. (2022). Why anti-racist education must include Asian American history. *Midwestern Educational Researcher, 34*(2). 205–220. https://scholarworks.bgsu.edu/mwer/vol34/iss2/7

Khoi the Poet. (2016, June 1). *Asian American history.* Youtube. https://www.youtube.com/watch?v=6pqVwrsGHtk

Kochhar, R., & Cilluffo, A. (2018). *Income inequality in the US is rising most rapidly among Asians.* Pew Research Center. https://mth101.com/wp-content/uploads/2020/04/Lab-13-Articles.pdf

Le, T. V., & Barboza-Wilkes, C. (2022). How the paradoxical treatment of Asian Americans as model minorities and perpetual foreigners shape their burnout experiences in local government. *Public Integrity, 24*(6), 550–572. https://doi.org/10.1080/10999922.2022.2071516

Lee, E. (2015). *The making of Asian America: A history* (Reprint ed.). Simon & Schuster.

Lee, P. (2020). Rejecting honorary whiteness: Asian Americans and the attack on race-conscious admissions. *Emory LJ, 70,* 1475. https://scholarlycommons.law.emory.edu/elj/vol70/iss7/3

Lee, S. J., Xiong, C., Pheng, L. M., & Vang, M. N. (2017). The model minority maze. *Journal of Southeast Asian American Education & Advancement, 12*(2), 1–20. https://www.jstor.org/stable/48684421

Liu-Countryman, J. (2017). The hard lessons of a model minority living in a racist world. In E. Dunbar, A. Blanco, D. A. Crèvecoeur-MacPhail, C. Munthe, M. Fingerle, & D. Brax (Eds.), *The psychology of hate crimes as domestic terrorism: U.S. and global issues: Assessment issues with victims and offenders* (pp. 103–118). Praeger/ABC-CLIO.

Louie-Poon, S., Idrees, S., Plesuk, T., Hilario, C., & Scott, S. D. (2022). Racism and the mental health of East Asian diasporas in North America: A scoping review. *Journal of Ment Health, 11,* 1-16. https://doi.org/10.1080/09638237.2022.2069715.

Luna, L. (n.d.). Asian Americans: Visibility and violence. UC Santa Barbara Humanities and Fine Arts. https://www.hfa.ucsb.edu/news-entries/2021/5/6/navigating-asian-american-visibility-and-violence

Makino, K. (2016). The framing discourses of 'honorary white' in the anti-apartheid movement in Japan. *IDE Discussion Paper*, 575.

Mineo, L. (2021, March 24). The scapegoating of Asian Americans. *The Harvard Gazette.* https://news.harvard.edu/gazette/story/2021/03/a-long-history-of-bigotry-against-asian-americans/

Mudambi, A. (2019). South Asian American discourses: Engaging the yellow peril-model minority dialectic. *Howard Journal of Communications, 30*(3), 284–298. https://doi.org/10.1080/10646175.2018.1491431

Noh, E. (2018). Terror as usual: The role of the model minority myth in Asian American women's suicidality. *Women & Therapy, 41*(3–4), 316–338. https://doi.org/10.1080/02703149.2018.1430360

Ong, A. (2006). *Neoliberalism as exception: Mutations in citizenship and sovereignty.* Duke University Press.

Park, G. C. (2011). Becoming a "model minority": Acquisition, construction and enactment of American identity for Korean immigrant students. *The Urban Review, 43*(5), 620–635. https://doi.org/10.1007/s11256-010-0164-8

Park, Y. J. (2008). White, honorary white, or non-white: Apartheid era constructions of Chinese. *Afro-Hispanic Review, 27*(1), 123–138. https://www.jstor.org/stable/23055227.

Park, M., Choi, Y., Yoo, H. C., Yasui, M., & Takeuchi, D. (2021). Racial stereotypes and Asian American youth paradox. *Journal of Youth and Adolescence, 50*(12), 2374–2393. https://doi.org/10.1007/s10964-021-01519-8

Petersen, W. (1966, January). Success story, Japanese-American style. *The New York Times Magazine*, 20–21, 33, 36, 38, 40–41, 43.

Ramakrishnan, K., & Ahmad, F. Z. (2014). State of Asian Americans and Pacific Islanders series: A multifaceted portrait of a growing population. https://cdn.americanprogress.org/wp-content/uploads/2014/04/AAPIReport-comp.pdf

Rodriguez-Operana, V. C., Mistry, R. S., & Chen, Y. J. (2017). Disentangling the myth: Social relationships and Filipino American adolescents' experiences of the model minority stereotype. *Asian American Journal of Psychology, 8*(1), 56–71. https://doi.org/10.1037/aap0000071

Sabharwal, M., Becerra, A., & Oh, S. (2022). From the Chinese Exclusion Act to the COVID-19 pandemic: A historical analysis of "otherness" experienced by Asian Americans in the United States. *Public Integrity, 24*(6), 535–549. https://doi.org/10.1080/10999922.2022.2120292

Said, E. W. (2003). *Orientalism.* Penguin.

Shih, K. Y., Chang, T. F., & Chen, S. Y. (2019). Impacts of the model minority myth on Asian American individuals and families: Social justice and critical race feminist perspectives. *Journal of Family Theory & Review, 11*(3), 412–428. https://doi.org/10.1111/jftr.12342

Sibango, B. (2022). Honorary whiteness as an ideological tool sustaining a hierarchical racial order and land expropriation in South Africa. *Filosofia Theoretica: Journal of African Philosophy, Culture and Religions, 11*(3), 51–66. https://hdl.handle.net/10520/ejc-filosofia_v11_n3_a5.

Subramanian, T. (2019, July 25). Demystifying internalized oppression: Being the "model minority" isn't a compliment: How internalizing the model minority does more harm than good. *The Inclusion Solution.*    https://theinclusionsolution.me/demystifying-internalized-oppression-being-the-model-minority-isnt-a-compliment-how-internalizing-the-model-minority-myth-does-more-harm-than-good-asian-american/.

Trieu, M. M., & Lee, H. C. (2018). Asian Americans and internalized racial oppression: Identified, reproduced, and dismantled. *Sociology of Race and Ethnicity, 4*(1), 67–82. https://doi.org/10.1177/23326492177257.

Tuan, M. (1998). *Forever foreigners or honorary whites?: The Asian ethnic experience today*. Rutgers University Press.

Walton, J., & Truong, M. (2023). A review of the model minority myth: understanding the social, educational and health impacts. *Ethnic and Racial Studies, 46*(3), 391–419. https://doi.org/10.1080/01419870.2022.2121170

Wang, C., Wang, J., & Lin, M. (2021). COVID-19 and Asian phobia: Anti-Asian racism and model minority myth. *New Waves, 24*(2), I–VI.

Whaley, A. L., & Noel, L. T. (2013). Academic achievement and behavioral health among Asian American and African American adolescents: Testing the model minority and inferior minority assumptions. *Social Psychology of Education, 16*(1), 23–43. https://doi.org/10.1007/s11218-012-9206-2

Wing, J. Y. (2007). Beyond black and white: The model minority myth and the invisibility of Asian American students. *The Urban Review, 39*(4), 455–487. https://doi.org/10.1007/s11256-007-0058-6

Wu, C., Qian, Y., & Wilkes, R. (2021). Anti-Asian discrimination and the Asian-white mental health gap during COVID-19. *Ethnic and Racial Studies, 44*(5), 819–835. https://doi.org/10.1080/01419870.2020.1851739

Wu, L., & Nguyen, N. (2022). From yellow peril to model minority and back to yellow peril. *Aera Open, 8*(1), 1–10., https://doi.org/10.1177/23328584211067796

Xu, J., & Lee, J. C. (2013). The marginalized "model" minority: An empirical examination of the racial triangulation of Asian Americans. *Social Forces, 91*(4), 1363–1397. https://doi.org/10.1093/sf/sot049

Yi Borromeo, V. 2018. *A phenomenological inquiry into the racialized experiences of Southeast Asian American community college students*. [Doctoral dissertation] University of Denver. https://digitalcommons.du.edu/etd/1437

Yim, J. Y. (2009). *"Being an Asian American male is really hard actually"*: *Cultural psychology of Asian American masculinities and psychological well-being*. University of Michigan.

Yip, T., Cheah, C. S., Kiang, L., & Hall, G. C. N. (2021). Rendered invisible: Are Asian Americans a model or a marginalized minority? *American Psychologist, 76*(4), 575–581. https://doi.org/10.1037/amp0000857

Young, A. V. (2009). Honorary whiteness. *Asian Ethnicity, 10*(2), 177–185. https://doi.org/10.1080/14631360902906862

Zhou, M. (2012). *Asians in America: The paradox of" the model minority" and" the perpetual foreigner"*. University of Saskatchewan.

Zou, L. X., & Cheryan, S. (2022). Diversifying neighborhoods and schools engender perceptions of foreign cultural threat among white Americans. *Journal of Experimental Psychology: General, 151*(5), 1115–1131. https://doi.org/10.1037/xge0001115

# Chapter 3

# Racialized Gender's Rupturing of Asian American Identities and Relationships

*Jessica ChenFeng and Lana Kim*

The relationship we have to, and our experience of gender is complex. Especially for the Asian American person and identity, there are countless intersections to country of origin, history, generation, and family to culture, religion, and experience of race and gender within dominant U.S. society. This chapter discusses these intersections of Asian American identity and gender and is merely one of many ways to make sense of who we are and how we connect to others and ourselves.

Even as we engaged in research for this chapter, we experienced what is felt by many—that our encounters related to gender can come with so much pain and trauma and continue to create or fuel ongoing stress in ourselves, our families, and relationships. Larger societal discourse on gender contributes to the challenge of having a meaningful exploration of and discussion around gender. Much of this has similar undertones to conversations about race where terms such as privilege, oppression, power, and marginalization activate all kinds of feelings in people. It is not hard to resort to an us vs. them, women vs. men posture.

It is important to develop critical consciousness about ourselves from our social locations AND humbly recognize that the systems of power and oppression within which we all reside are harmful to all genders and relationships. Patriarchy, in all its forms, does not only hurt women but is hurtful to all genders and our capacities to see one another as full, whole human beings. The work we do in our own lives and with our clients is not only about increasing critical consciousness on a cognitive level but also developing awareness about our internal processes and visceral relational dynamics.

This chapter is in the first part of the book (contextualizing silence and invisibility) because while there are certainly narratives of resilience and strength, our racialized gendered realities have often been connected to our experiences of silence and invisibility. We will first approach the conversation by offering some key historical and contextual background. Then we will share clinical concepts that have transformed our understanding of how to theorize and approach gender in clinical contexts.

DOI: 10.4324/9781003321590-5

## Asian American Gender Discourses Across Time and Place

We hope that this book is highlighting the significance of knowing and understanding our legacies and experiences of migration. No matter how, when, or why our families migrated, the experiences of displacement and rupture have generational effects. The sociopolitical contexts of that time and place shaped the ancestors and elders who left. We hold curiosity about how gender was understood and experienced in countries of origin at the time of departure. What happens when these individuals and families relocate to North American lands and contexts? What happens to the perspectives and relational patterns related to gender? What global and local histories have taken place to give shape to the discourse and imaginations that the U.S. has about Asian American identity? How does the dynamic interplay with a shifting racial and sociopolitical context continue to transform Asian American identity, relationships, and family life? These are the dialogues to consider as we continue the conversation.

### Migration and Generation

Because post-migration life in the U.S. is often about survival, it is not typical for the first few generations of Asian Americans to talk about pre-migration histories and family contexts. As mentioned in Chapter 1, sometimes the experience of loss, trauma, and grief can be an understandable reason that the first generation, whether intentionally or not, does not want to revisit memories of the land, life, and relationships left behind. They may also not see the value or purpose in doing so because their focus is on trying to make it in the U.S. and the future they are creating for themselves and their families. An all-too-common unintended consequence of this intergenerational process is *disenfranchised grief* (Doka, 1989). This is grief that for whatever reason cannot be acknowledged, felt, responded to, or socially supported. Perhaps being in a state of survival required a response of repression to keep vulnerable feelings of sadness and loss at bay. Or even though the grief is felt from tense family dynamics, there might not be any tangible context to make sense of it. Consequently, next-generation adult children might internalize, personalize, and experience an exacerbation of this inherited grief and trauma and wonder, "What's wrong with me? Why am I having such a hard time if my first-generation parents seem fine?" because of missing a contextual and historical perspective.

### The First Generation Context

The first generation bears a lot given what they endured through being uprooted and displaced. In *Asian American Sexual Politics*, Taiwanese American sociologist Rosalind Chou discusses how it "can be difficult [for first generation Asian Americans] to balance the 'old world' and the 'new world'" (Chou, 2010, p. 52) when it comes to gender roles and expectations. Their home countries may have had certain scripts about gender, and finding themselves in a new country with unfamiliar gender discourses can make parenting bicultural children especially challenging. Thus, it is helpful to know the influences, ideas, and discourses about gender one brings from their country of origin. While Asian countries might share some similar social, political, and religious contexts that shape the construction of gender, it is important to not make assumptions. Instead, we need to explore and understand each Asian American family's legacy, the intersections of multiple Asian heritages, and how individuals and families negotiate gender.

Many Asian cultures share the ethos of kinship which serves as the organizing principle under which gender becomes more visible. Kinship is about how members are placed into social groups, including the family household and what their responsibilities and obligations are to one another (Dube, 1988). With the long histories of all Asian countries (and "country" is not always the best identifier as ethnic groups do not necessarily align with changing political borders), the influence of indigenous traditions, religions (Hindu, Buddhist, Islamic, Christian, etc.), European colonization, geography, and wars give shape to the landscape of kinship and gender. There are a variety of kinship systems across Asia, including patrilineal, matrilineal, and bilateral (Dube, 1997). Exploring clients' inheritance of kinship models would be another informative part of the assessment.

For example, Confucianism has broadly influenced a number of East and Southeast Asian cultural systems. These include China, Japan, Korea, and Vietnam, as well as cultures and nations influenced by the Chinese, including Taiwan, Singapore, and Malaysia (Lee, 2010). Though the concept of gender in Confucian philosophy is complex, what is significant to highlight here is the lingering legacy and emphasis on patrilineage and women's relationship to men that can present in traditional cultural systems:

> Women are the ones who follow others; when they are young they follow their fathers and elder brothers, when they are married they follow their husbands, and when their husbands die they follow their sons.
>
> (*Liji*, "*Jiaotesheng*" chapter, as cited in Rosenlee, 2023)

While some Asian cultures inherit a patriarchal structure, it is important to not assume that Asian American clients align with or practice these values. It is helpful, however, to understand and explore the ways that Asian kinship systems are historical and generational, and not simply static and fixed family values.

Another relevant concept for the first generation is this the idea that "social relations at peak times of migration have an impact on contemporary social relations" (Lung, 2023). The point in time within history in which the first generation leaves their country-of-origin becomes the time capsule that determines which values, relational understandings, cultural, political, and gendered realities get deeply embedded and embodied. It is not uncommon for Asian migrants to the U.S. to have more traditional or "outdated" schema than their contemporaries who did not experience migration because they missed out on the ways that their home countries continued to evolve and modernize. There is something valid about wanting to hold on to cultural values and norms as the first generation sought to establish family life in a new and foreign place. However, the implicit gendered kinship systems can be imposed on the second generation and contribute to cultural clashes and intergenerational tensions.

### Second Generation and Beyond

The second+ generation Asian American experience of gender is characterized by many layers of tension: bicultural, intergenerational, and racial. These tensions can be about the way that gender was performed, taught, or spoken about in the family in light of the larger American discourses absorbed from the dominant culture. The tensions are also about collectivistic kinship values of the family while trying to manage and engage in Western individualistic spaces. Rather than viewing the tension as one value system versus the other, or that Asian Americans have to choose between opposing ethics, we believe Asian Americans straddle cultures as they navigate their bicultural racialized identities. For example:

- "Girls/women should be modest and respectful" and "girls/women should be strong and speak up"
- "Obligation to and honoring your family and parents is important" and "a queer young person should be proud and stand up for themselves"
- "Men lead their families and take charge of their homes" and "Asian men are passive and not capable of leading teams"

It is important for therapists to be curious about and explore these bicultural, intergenerational, and racial realities and not assume that seemingly disparate discourses are mutually exclusive. Rather, how do we support clients in sitting with and making sense of these tensions?

### Binary Constructions of Gender

Asian cultures have rich and diverse histories of gender and sexualities. Much of this was reordered and narrowed as a result of Western imperialism (Loos, 2009) and the influence of male-centric, hierarchical religions (Peletz, 2006). Consequently, Asian migrants brought to the U.S. a binary understanding of gender; this, along with the strong Asian American value of *conformity to norms*

(Kim, Li & Ng., 2005), and a male hegemonic U.S. landscape, creates a context that is oppressive to Asian Americans whose identities and lives are outside of this binary. Post-migration, many Asian American families are influenced by the unyielding Christian white cisheteropatriarchal cultural history of the U.S. Asian cultural legacies of gender along with dominant U.S. discourses create an especially hostile reality for anything that challenges the gender binary: identities, relationships, and ways of being that are not socially sanctioned expectations of male/female, masculine/feminine.

While this chapter primarily wrestles with the construction of Asian American gender identity, certainly gender and sexuality are intricately connected. We encourage readers to further explore these intersectional discourses for themselves and clients. The absence of conversations on sexuality in the Asian American family system, the historical ways Asian American sexuality has been omitted and rejected, give shape to a longing for greater understanding, honest conversation, and intra/interpersonal healing. This is a growing area of research and conversation.

### Asian American Racialization Across U.S. History

Because Asian American history has been omitted and is still not reliably included or taught as part of U.S. history, all of us, including Asian Americans, are disconnected from a historical contextual understanding of the long legacy of racialization. There is so much more than we can highlight here, but we offer some ways to make sense of what has given shape to the construction of present-day Asian American femininities and masculinities.

We resonate with the perspective of media law scholar and attorney Michael Park, who in his article on the legal and historical perspectives of Asian American masculinity, emphasizes that "racialized masculinity is shaped by historical, political and cultural forces... racialized masculinity is also constructed, rather than found. Immigration policies and its implications on Asian masculinity present histories to be explored" (Park, 2013, p. 6). We believe this is true across Asian American masculinities and femininities—that gender is always racialized and that race/racism is always gendered. Race and gender processes are intertwined and thus are the effects on individuals and families.

#### Exploitation of Labor and a Threat to Be Extinguished

Since the first large wave of Asian migration in the late 1800s, Asian Americans have been exploited for their labor, especially during times of U.S. financial growth. With a settler colonial mentality of domination, the New World was developing and laborers were needed to build the railroad. Chinese workers could be purchased for two-thirds the cost of their white counterparts and so began an anti-Asian/Chinese sentiment because white laborers' jobs were threatened. This pattern has been repeated across U.S. history, and the implications have been deadly. In 1982, Chinese American Vincent Chin was out with friends in Detroit, Michigan, celebrating his upcoming wedding. Two white male autoworkers beat Chin to death because they were angry over the loss of American auto work to the rise of Japanese carmakers.

This has been a painful and persistent way that Asian Americans have been racialized: that we are "good workers" because we are experienced as compliant and hard-working. Yet we are never accepted or belong; instead, we are perceived as a threat to be extinguished. This led to a number of exclusionary laws targeting Chinese men (not allowed to testify against whites, not able to become citizens, anti-miscegenation laws, not allowed to form their own families); these practices "would limit job opportunities, prevent family formations, and effectively emasculate Asian men" (Park, 2013, p. 7).

Across these capitalism-fueled pressures, Asian men were racialized as predators of white women and in the 1920s, 400 white men attacked a Filipino dance hall after the publication of a photo showing a white teenage girl and Filipino man embracing (Lee, 2019). We invite you to consider the centuries-long racialized double bind that many Asian Americans have endured, giving shape to a persistent experience of feeling exploited and rejected. When we humanize the Asian migrant and consider their plight in leaving/being forced out of a home country, no matter what the sociopolitical condition was, we imagine their dreams and hopes of having their basic needs met, to be able to provide for their transnational and new families. The tension of holding on to hope amid Asian bodies being the target of hate—what a profound resilience and strength that lives in our bodies and has been inherited across generations.

### Exclusion and Dehumanization

Using Asian Americans to serve white capitalism, then resenting and hating them, serves to maintain white power and racial purity. However, many of us have not had the opportunity to learn this history in order to contextualize our experiences and can easily internalize the feelings as "something is wrong with me that I feel this way" or "how come people treat me this way, I must not fit in."

Because through the 19th century Asian men were barred from having basic rights, they were forced to create communities among themselves, learning traditionally "women's duties" such as cooking and cleaning. In the early 1900s, the population of Asian women was very low (Okihiro, 1994), and many were relegated to work as prostitutes. This further perpetuated ideas about Asian men being effeminate and they were "constructed as impotent and their women as 'whores'" (Chou, 2010, p. 26). Asian bodies were acknowledged and known only by way of their subservience to white supremacy.

Asians were further dehumanized by affiliating them with bringing in "filth from the orient." Whether Asian bodies or Asian food, they were characterized as "uncivilized savages" because U.S. colonizers did not know how to make sense of another way of being outside of their narrow white hegemonic masculine frameworks of manifest destiny. Microaggressions perpetuating the forever foreigner stereotype ("where are you from?" "your English is good"), Asian fetishism (attraction to "the exotic" or to the "submissive") and regular encounters of outright racism remind us that we have never been accepted as "American" and that we are not seen and known for who we really are. The thousands of documented hate incidents against Asian Americans (stopaapihate.org; harassment, physical harm, institutional discrimination, etc.) are part of this country's racist history.

### The Construction of Asian American Racialized Gender

We touched upon some of these themes of Asian American racialization to highlight the significance of white hegemony, migration, and policy in the construction of racialized gender. These intersect with the Asian cultural kinship systems our own families inherited and passed on across the generations. A third-order lens (McDowell, Knudson-Martin, & Bermudez, 2019) compels us to consider how all these systems influence our relationship with our own Asian American gendered identity. How do they shape our relationships with family within Asian American contexts? How do they affect our relationships with communities outside of our racial/ethnic spaces? How do they frame and posture our capacities to connect relationally in meaningful and mutual ways?

As we consider ourselves and clients along the spectrum of well-being and mental health, it is important to ask: In what ways might one's experience of depression, anxiety, relationship distress, and other barriers to hoped-for functioning be intertwined with the construction of racialized gender? Whether conscious or not, communities of color are familiar with living under a *white gaze*—the everyday reality of living, breathing, functioning in response to a white dominant world. From every possible angle, we internalize messages about what is right, ideal, best, preferred, good, healthy, and normal, all of which are normed by white standards. Internalizing this white gaze means that our thoughts and behaviors align with whiteness' definitions of who we should be for them, which is why trying to live up to the model minority myth can be so exhausting and lead to symptoms of depression and anxiety.

Another theme is the intergenerational inheritance of *kinship values and expectations*. Among the many ways that families "teach" their children about how to be in the world, messages about kinship values and gender roles and expectations can be some of the strongest. Becoming a "good" daughter or son, wife or husband, has everything to do with family, community, honor, and generational legacy and can elicit deep feelings of pride or shame. These processes can be so profound that they are embodied before they can be cognitively understood.

With these often competing discourses (the white gaze alongside kinship values/expectations), we as Asian Americans find ourselves living in persistent states of *negotiation, tension, and wrestling* with identity and relationships. For example, one's family-of-origin cultural values may feel counter to white American discourses; workplace expectations of gender may not align with how one wishes to be known.

### Asian American Women and Femininity

With the longstanding U.S. history of objectifying Asian American women's bodies, it makes sense that there is much tension within Asian American women's relationships to their own bodies: Perceptions of beauty as defined by colonizers (Euro-centric features of light skin, large eyes, high cheekbones) along with how Asian women are expected to present (cute and youthful) in order to fit into the ideals defined by a white gaze of Asian American women. While women of any racial background may experience pressure to fit into societally defined internalized standards of beauty, for Asian American women, this can be exacerbated by the fear and pain of societal and familial rejection. Within patriarchal systems, Asian mothers' implicit duties traditionally include ensuring their daughter's ability to compete in the cis hetero marriage arena, which often means socializing them to racialized and cultural feminine standards. When daughters reject this set of expectations regarding femininity (appearance, body, temperament, presentation, skillset, etc.), mothers may respond with criticism and shame which fuels harmful generational cycles of internalized sexism and racism that result in relational disconnection. Furthermore, the pressure to conform to these oppressive standards can get reified by one's partner or in-laws in the cis hetero marital context.

In and out of the domestic context, Asian American women have to negotiate tensions across multiple relational systems—some that center hierarchy, others collaboration, some that champion women's empowerment, and others that expect traditional racialized depictions of Asian female submission. Women who live this daily experience of shifting between spaces can develop a competence per se around code-switching and bridge-building, but this can also be exhausting and confusing.

This internal wrestling that Asian American women unconsciously do is rarely acknowledged or seen. It is worth exploring the ways that Asian American women's positionality in relationships and social contexts are negotiated day to day and the implications on personal health and identity. When a therapist sees, identifies, gives voice, and validates the socioemotional contextual load that Asian American women bear, it can be profoundly healing.

*The Construction of Asian American Men and Masculinity*

What does it mean to be an Asian American man? So many discourses speak into the assumptions and expectations: a dutiful son, a privileged preferred son, a chauvinistic husband, a committed dedicated worker, physically agile, nerdy and humble, a deceitful manipulative gangster, a stoic father. Mixed messages are sent and media portrayals of these racist stereotypes are essentializing. Asian American men are privileged in traditional familial and cultural systems of patrilineage, but marginalized as men in white dominant society without options to move up the ladder that do not involve colluding with dominant power practices. That is, even if Asian men inherit patriarchal lineages, the unidimensional narratives about their patriarchy are reductionistic and rob them of any chance of being understood, acknowledged, and seen. This leaves them struggling to find ways to resolve grief and pain; their microscopic presence in our social imagination can lead to further shrinking away or contrastingly, to puffing up—an exhibition of hypermasculinity in order to compensate for the inequities of racialized gender (J. Chu, personal communication, February 14, 2024).

Whether in Asian cultural contexts or within the dominant white U.S. society, boys and men are not typically socialized to be attuned to their emotional states or that of others. They might even be discouraged from it or ridiculed because it is perceived to be "girly" or "feminine." There can be unspoken costs in pursuing the desire or expectation to fulfill kinship roles of husband, father, and son, in family life and to have a successful career outside. The weighty cultural gender scripts prescribed to Asian men about their familial duties mixed with the racist tropes about them create a high pressure context. The delegitimization of emotion and lack of awareness around their own stress affect their ability to attune to the emotions of others which can lead to cycles of relational disconnection and exacerbate questions around self-worth. It is not hard to understand the external and internal burdens of pursuing outward success in order to fulfill family duties and racialized expectations.

Researchers are now intentionally studying the connections between shame, addiction, and gendered racism for Asian American men. The pain of not being able to meet white hegemonic ideals of masculinity is associated with greater shame, which then intensifies depressive symptoms and has implications for feeling even greater shame toward the family, which is then connected with greater alcohol use (Keum & Choi, 2023). For men living out these cycles, the intrapersonal pain is profound as are the effects on their significant relationships.

For the Asian American men who find themselves in therapy, there may be an earnestness in wanting to grow and experience healing for themselves and their relationships, especially in disentangling from the harms of patriarchy. But therapists must not equate Asian American men's symptoms of patriarchy with that of white men. When Asian American men perform patriarchal values, this needs to be conceptualized in relation to their racialized gendered pain of being delegitimized in their worth, by U.S. society. We need to validate and affirm that Asian American men deserve to be seen and visible in a life where they have been historically erased and obsolete, without having to adopt superficial "power over" practices that harm their relationships. Unless their racialized gendered pain is made visible, movement toward mutuality in their relationships will be inauthentic.

## Engaging with Racialized Gender in the Clinical Space

There are so many ways that we can engage a clinical conversation around gender. We believe that therapists are not neutral participants in the therapeutic process. We come with our own lived experiences and sociocultural political contexts that shape our values and perspectives about what it means to best support our clients. With this in mind, there are two clinical concepts we have found helpful and want to invite as tools for framing and assessing Asian Americans' relationships to racialized gender. Rather than this chapter being about how to "do therapy" in a particular way, our hope is that the information here allows us to see how critically important it is to make sense of racialized gender as it connects to self, family, history, and sociocultural context. As discussed in the introduction, *third-order thinking* is foundational in this book. McDowell, Knudson-Martin, and Bermudez (2019) offer some general principles about how to facilitate third-order change. It requires us as therapists to:

(1) take a metaview of ourselves and the families with whom we work as acting within systems of systems
(2) integrate our understanding of societal systems and power into treatment models, and
(3) invite clients to view their own lives from metaperspectives that assist them in solving problems and expanding possibilities for organizing relationships (McDowell, Knudson-Martin, & Bermudez, 2019, p. 14).

We discuss these two clinical concepts, *contextual differentiation* and *relational flow of power*, highlighting the third-order nature of applying these in two cases. A key component of the posture we take is being comfortable moving into spaces of tension, embracing the both/and breaking out of society's zero-sum pull to pick one way of being. We also share some personal reflections about our own journeys of what it has looked like to expand possibilities in our own experiences of being racialized East Asian North American women.

### Contextual Differentiation

One way of facilitating third-order change is through supporting the development of *contextual differentiation* in ourselves and our clients. In my early years

(JCF), I was trained under a Bowenian Family Systems therapist and was drawn to the theory's concepts of differentiation and autonomy/interdependence. When I began working with primarily Asian American clients, it was evident that these concepts required expansion or some kind of third-order reframe (at the time I had not been introduced to third-order thinking). If we understand individual differentiation as the growing capacity to distinguish between our own thoughts and feelings from that of another person, or of our families, then contextual differentiation is about being able to discern what we feel, think, and sense and in what ways this might be shaped and influenced by larger societal discourses. Being able to contextually differentiate can significantly shift an Asian American person's experience of themselves and the relationships they hold dear.

Ruth is a 58-year-old first-generation Indonesian American woman who is experiencing stress in caring for both her aging and ailing mother, who lives with them, and their two young adult children also living at home. Her first-generation Indonesian American husband is a few years older and just retired from working for the U.S. Postal Service. Ruth is in the last few years of her career as a labor and delivery nurse. Current stressors include her own health issues of unknown cause, guilt about considering placing her mother in a nursing facility, her husband's overbearing presence at home, and workplace communication stress.

Moving toward increasing contextual differentiation would involve walking with Ruth to unpack the discourses around gender that have shaped how she understands herself in relationship:

- What does it mean to be a good mom, wife, daughter, nurse? Taking the time to explore the histories related to these identities.
- What has she internalized about the personal, familial, and social consequences for deviating from these scripts/discourses? What does this mean about a mom, wife, etc.?
- Are there experiences that stand out (moments of embarrassment, shame, etc.) that have led to fear or trauma around this racialized gender identity? For example, witnessing her own mother be shamed by her paternal grandmother for not being a good wife/mother for choosing to work so much outside of the home.

In unpacking these discourses, it is important to support Ruth in giving voice to how these discourses are not only personal or familial but also racial, embedded in generational historical contexts. The hope is to shift from a first- or second-order lens (something is wrong with me, my family system is unhealthy) to a third-order perspective (curiosity and awareness of how the larger systems influence who she is and feels pressured to be).

The therapist can support Ruth in thinking and feeling beyond her immediate social context (the heaviness of family and home life, weighty workplace dynamics) to exploring different metaperspectives. Are there Asian American women in her world that intrigue her because they are attempting to find solutions that deviate from cultural norms or racial expectations? How are they doing so, and how does Ruth experience them in their venturing into alternative scripts?

Increasing contextual differentiation does not necessarily mean that a client arrives at a conclusion about who they are and can clearly delineate themselves from family and from context. This is a possibility, but change is more nuanced. We aim to support clients to develop contextual differentiation that enables them to better sit with the tension of multiple discourses, understand the journey around where they came from, have more curiosity around their own process of balancing competing expectations, hold less self-judgment, and exercise more freedom to reject the perceived critique from others.

### Relational Flow of Power

Another useful clinical concept we highlight comes from Socio-Emotional Relationship Therapy (SERT), a framework for couples therapy (Knudson-Martin, 2023). Being able to *identify the relational flow of power* has become a critically important tool in our work with clients because we believe the way SERT centers mutuality is something worth pursuing and expanding in people's relationships.

When we consider Asian American identity, power is typically understood from a structural perspective and related to one's social location. Some Asian American clients may not experience themselves as having much power in U.S. society from the perspective of their racialized experiences of being invisible, not being perceived as trustworthy/credible, which renders them without much agency and influence. Asian Americans may also buy into the model minority stereotype, whereby "making it" is measured by class status and upward mobility. This barometer is disconnected from any painful cultural legacies and can give the false impression of superiority to other Asian Americans or other people of color. The complex intersections of racialization and internalized racism show up in the flow of power within Asian American relationships.

SERT conceptualizes power as a relational attribute (as opposed to a static personal characteristic) and as a process *between* people. This process between people (or the relational flow of power) can be made more visible by exploring and observing "how the experience of being attended to and the ability to influence the relationship moves from one to another or accumulates toward one person or group" (Knudson-Martin, 2023, p. 63). The way this flow of power moves within relationships is usually unconscious to those involved, and the person with more relational power is especially unaware. The intention of SERT is to support the couple toward increased mutuality in their relationship. Here are some helpful questions to ask to identify the relational flow of power (Knudson-Martin, 2023, p. 341):

- How much personal, interpersonal, and institutional power does each client experience as a result of their societal positions?
- To what extent is each person equally able to express and attain personal interests/goals?
- To what extent do each expect to define what is "real"?
- To what extent does each person organize around what matters to the other(s)?
- Whose interests are most reflected in "shared" decisions?
- Whose interests and schedule organize daily schedules and routines?
- How are differences in opinion handled?
- Who is more likely to accommodate the other person(s)?
- Does accommodation often occur automatically without anything being said?
- Does one person's sense of competence, optimism, or well-being seem to come at the expense of the other's physical or emotional health?
- Does the relationship support the economic viability of each person?

What we have learned is that in the clinical encounter, it does not necessarily work to simply tell or ask clients about the flow of power. Because these dynamics are unconscious, addressing power head on with clients without efforts to socioculturally attune to their socioemotional experience with power, will leave them feeling blamed, criticized, or misunderstood. This will present as resistance or disengagement in the therapeutic process. It is also very likely that Asian American clients are unfamiliar with ideas of power and/or have static understandings of it. As such, the process of change does not simply happen by engaging in overt conversations about power.

We are not delving into the details of how to practice SERT, but highlighting how we might work with the SERT concept of relational flow of power as a way Asian Americans can negotiate the racialized gendered dynamics of power. We invite you to consider with us that it may be an unrealistic goal to experience mutuality in every relational dynamic. However, it is possible that by growing in contextual differentiation, we become more capable of identifying the flow of power in our relationships, and thereby have increased consciousness to empower where and how we negotiate relational power.

Jamie and Lisa are a queer couple, both in their early 30s. Jamie is a second-generation Korean American and Lisa is second-/third-generation Taiwanese/Chinese. They sought out therapy because they have been having "communication issues" as they discuss their hopes of becoming parents. Jamie is the middle child in a middle-class Korean American family with strong affiliation with the

Korean Presbyterian Church, especially because her father has been the pastor of their family church for two decades. Lisa is the eldest in her family, which is nominally Buddhist, and grew up engaging in cultural practices, such as going to the temple and honoring ancestors. Though she would describe her family as not having any "strong religious values like Jamie's family," there were implicit messages about kinship values. For example, since Lisa was the firstborn grandchild, the paternal grandparents hoped that she would be a son. This implicitly shaped a lot of the expectations and socialization around Lisa's upbringing.

In their relational dynamic, Jamie feels as though Lisa has a stronger influence on when and how to become parents, and consequently, Jamie experiences the dynamic as unfair. This voicelessness in their partnership exacerbates a lot of the powerlessness she grew up feeling in her racialized gendered contexts. Lisa's parents wanted Lisa to grow up not feeling any less than as a girl granddaughter and taught her to speak up and express her opinions unapologetically. She feels irritated by Jamie's deferential relational posture and wants Jamie to be more expressive of her interests and preferences so they can "actually talk." This can be activating for Jamie because she has been shaped by her Korean Christian church culture with strong messages about the centrality of girls' modesty, submissive posture, and dutiful wifely skills for successful future partnership and to "honor God." It takes a lot for her to combat these messages and to access her own voice and preferences, thus "living up to" Lisa's expectations. It is possible that the flow of power goes to Lisa, even though she may not feel this way because in her mind, she is trying to empower Jamie. From a SERT perspective, Lisa's interests are centered and Jamie spends a lot of her energy trying to accommodate what Lisa wants and says, which is indicative of how the power flows in their partnership.

Part of supporting this couple toward increased mutuality is to increase their awareness of relational power dynamics through a socioemotionally attuned lens. For Jamie, this may mean exploring the racialized gender and religious discourses that set up fairly rigid ideas of the sort of woman she needed to become for the main purpose of becoming a wife and mother in the future. The hope is that instead of Jamie continuing to feel discouraged about her own "incapability of being a strong outspoken woman," she develops greater self-compassion because she can understand how constricting these overbearing racialized gendered discourses can be when reinforced across multiple contexts. In witnessing these conversations, Lisa develops contextual differentiation and socioemotional attunement to how differently they were socialized and has increased empathy for the many tensions Jamie has to negotiate. As the therapeutic process progresses with a SERT lens, Lisa becomes increasingly aware of how her more direct way of communicating can be experienced as patriarchal and is surprised to realize that how she communicates could be adding stress to Jamie. In becoming more aware of the flow of power in their dynamic—when, how, and why

Lisa's actions and words have such a significant impact on Jamie—Lisa starts to practice and learn how to adapt her communication style and the skill of checking in and deferring to Jamie. Over time, Jamie learns to trust Lisa's efforts and trust in her own voice because Lisa is consistently demonstrating that Jamie's needs matter and that Lisa is learning how to better attune because of Jamie.

### Our Personal Experiences

I (JCF) grew up in East Asian Christian church contexts (Taiwanese, Chinese, Korean) in an era where white evangelicalism shaped a lot of the Asian immigrant church's messages about gender and women's roles, identities, and pursuits. Becoming a good wife and mother was of utmost importance, and this also meant knowing how to "submit to a husband" because there were right roles and positions for women and men in the home and at church. In my own family context, the patriarchal flow of power was evident and the Asian church cultural dynamics reinforced this by validating women when they were good at cooking and serving and men when they were strong leaders. Outside of these ethnic religious enclaves, my experience as an Asian American racialized woman was consistent in setting after setting: I was mistaken for other Asian American women colleagues at every workplace, felt invisible because more often than not someone I had already met before would forget who I was, felt unknown outside of my accomplishments and outward contributions to academic/work environments, was objectified by men, including strangers, and became extremely adept at reading the room and others' expressions in order to please, appease, and not cause problems.

Though not an exhaustive list, the cumulative effect of these experiences fueled a perfectionistic tendency, a daily state of anxiety, and a fear of disappointing or letting others down. In a dysconscious way, I was pursuing the highest academic degree without any planned outcome, while partnered at that time with a man I was willing to follow, submit to, and defer to, and give up my career for.

It is not an exaggeration when I say that my education and years in therapy saved me and drastically shifted the trajectory of my life. Through the gift of participating in SERT research groups, exploring and dissecting my own therapeutic processes through writing, countless conversations with colleagues, mentors, and friends about our identities, wrestling with understanding and encountering power and marginalization, unpacking my own privilege and mistakes, I have had the benefit of growing in contextual differentiation, expanding my third order perspectives, and can better identify the flow of power in the relationships in my life. My husband and I have come a long way from our parents' generations in terms of trying to live out a more mutually supportive relationship, even as we have more to grow. Though racism and microaggressions will most likely continue to be an expected part of life, developing contextual differentiation has empowered me such that my inner world is less disrupted and I can identify the reasons for the flow of power in relationships, even if that means that sometimes I accept that in some dynamics, mutuality is not realistic. I can still be connected to myself, know my worth, and disentangle myself from the oppressive forces of racialized gender.

I (LK) grew up as the middle child with two brothers in a first-generation Korean Canadian family context. Our home was also a multigenerational one. But, since my dad grew up as an orphan, it was not his parents who lived with us as would be the cultural norm in patrilineal tradition. Instead, my maternal grandparents who immigrated to Canada the same year that I was born are the grandparent generation that lived with my family for the majority of my brothers and my upbringing. My late halmoni (maternal grandmother) played a major role in raising my brothers and me, and three younger female cousins who were like sisters to us. She was regarded as the Kim family matriarch and she was deeply beloved and respected, including by our family's Korean church community. My halmoni was known for her exceptional cooking and boundless generosity, so our family frequently hosted large family and church gatherings, where I learned by example that a primary function of my role was to serve others. This, in combination with my birth order position as the eldest, cisgender female cousin among the residing familial subgroup, influenced my gender role expectations and socialization. I received the most validation and affirmation when I was living up to the culturally defined tasks of caring for others and carrying the relational responsibility for managing emotions in relationships.

The elder generation subscribed to patrilineal values, and this was demonstrated in how they moved through their daily life. Because of the position and respect my maternal grandparents held in the family, their beliefs subsequently passed down to my generation. My haraboji held latent male power that was seen in the way that my halmoni and her daughters noticed and oriented around his needs and actively protected his patriarchal identity. He had the privilege to freely express his anger, and it was my halmoni's responsibility to accommodate and manage his emotions. Yet, even though my halmoni, mom, and aunts all demonstrated traditional Korean gender ethics, they also performed a particular version of feminized, cultural roles that defied the stereotypic notion of submissive or deferential. My halmoni was the person who everyone turned to for guidance and direction, and she was respected for her quiet strength, wisdom, and humility. My mom and aunts told us of how she was credited for pulling the family out of poverty and devastation post-Korean war by her savvy business sense and determination when my grandfather lost his accumulated wealth during the war that left him emotionally and psychologically traumatized. My mom also told me how my halmoni had convinced her father who was a teacher in the village to teach her how to read and write despite her paternal grandmother forbidding her education as a girl in 1930s Korea. As a woman, halmoni modeled the pursuit of personal power and raised daughters who were strong, industrious, courageous, and capable. But, she also maintained a cultural commitment to upholding male privilege. Growing up with this dualism, as a bicultural person who was born and socialized to western Canadian cultural norms, I became highly vigilant and attuned to the gender rules prescribed in different contexts and code-switched accordingly. I stepped back in deference when it was expected and stepped forward with assertion when needed.

However, similar to Jessica, my involvement in SERT research groups with Carmen Knudson-Martin and Douglas Huenergardt during doctoral education really catalyzed a paradigm shift in terms of my understanding of gender power dynamics through a socioemotionally attuned lens. The Circle of Care (Knudson-Martin, 2013) processes that facilitate mutually supporting relationships gave me a tangible framework and language to discuss and name my visceral experiences of the flow of power as it relates to gender and other social identities. It also gave me a clinical lens to help challenge the structural inequities that are harmful for clients' relationships. Through my continued research, writing, and clinical practice I have numerous examples confirming my belief that using a socioemotionally attuned lens to interrupting the flow of power is critical to creating third-order change in the therapeutic process.

## Conclusion

In a chapter like this, it can feel like there is so much left unaddressed, so many realities and possibilities around how racialized gender is lived out in the lives of Asian Americans. This content is deep and multifaceted and the implications are serious and real. Deep grief and pain is an appropriate response. Too often Asian American racialized gender is invisible and glossed over. To truly bear witness to our experiences—the unique struggles of all Asian American genders—moves us in the direction of being acknowledged and becoming more seen and known. This is the path to hope and healing that is grounded in honest recognition and transformation.

## Reflection Questions

### Questions for Therapist

- What are the implicit or explicit values your family has around gender? How might this have intersected with your journey of becoming a therapist?
- What is your sense of how the U.S. dominant society views Asian American men? Women? How does your local training/clinical/academic setting view Asian American men/women?

- In what ways does your own racialized gender identity show up and get responded to by your current work and personal contexts? How does this affect you?
- Are there peers that you can connect with about these experiences?

### Questions for Therapy

- Can you tell me about the values—implicit or explicit—your family has around gender? For example, are girls and boys treated/valued similarly? Are there distinct roles that each parent plays?
- What does it mean to be a good son? Daughter? Wife? Husband?
- What are some tensions you feel about some of these roles or values from your family of origin in relation to what you've learned or absorbed growing up in the U.S.?
- What is your sense of how the U.S. dominant society views Asian American men? Women? Does this show up in your life? How so?

# References

Chou, R. (2010). *Asian American sexual politics: The construction of race, gender, and sexuality.* [Doctoral dissertation, Texas A&M University]. https://oaktrust.library.tamu.edu/bitstream/handle/1969.1/ETD-TAMU-2010-05-7870/CHOU-DISSERTATION_rev.pdf?sequence=5&isAllowed=y

Doka, K. (1989). *Disenfranchised grief: Recognizing hidden sorrow.* Lexington Books.

Dube, L. (1988). On the construction of gender: Hindu girls in patrilineal India. *Economic and Political Weekly, 23,* 18.

Dube, L. (1997). *Women and kinship: Comparative perspectives on gender in South and South-East Asia.* UNU Press.

Lee, E. (2019). *America for Americans: a history of xenophobia in the United States* (1st ed.). Basic Books.

Lee, M. H. (2010). Confucian traditions in modern East Asia: Their destinies and prospects. *Oriens Extremus, 49,* 237–247.

Keum, B. T., & Choi, A. Y. (2023). Gendered racism, family and external shame, depressive symptoms, and alcohol use severity among Asian American men. *Cultural Diversity and Ethnic Minority Psychology, 29*(2), 259.

Kim, B. K., Li, L. C., & Ng, G. F. (2005). The Asian American values scale--multidimensional: Development, reliability, and validity. *Cultural Diversity and Ethnic Minority Psychology, 11*(3), 187.

Knudson-Martin, C. (2013). Why power matters: Creating a foundation of mutual support in couple relationships. *Family Process, 52*(1), 5–18. https://doi.org/10.1111/FAMP.12011

Loos, T. (2009). Transnational histories of sexualities in Asia. *The American Historical Review, 114*(5), 1309–1324.

Lung, S. (2023, April 28). *Taiwanese churches in diaspora and ethnic identity formation* [workshop]. Multiple belongings in transpacific Christianities: Christian faith and Asian migration to the U.S. https://caac.ptsem.edu/dr-shirley-lung-taiwanese-churches-in-diaspora-and-ethnic-identity-formation/

McDowell, T., Knudson-Martin, C., & Bermudez, J. M. (2019). Third-order thinking in family therapy: Addressing social justice across family therapy practice. *Family Process*, *58*(1), 9–22. https://doi.org/10.1111/famp.12383

Okihiro, G. (1994). *Margins and mainstreams: Asians in American history and culture.* University of Washington Press, 1994.

Park, M. (2013). Asian American masculinity eclipsed: A legal and historical perspective of emasculation through U.S. immigration practices. *The Modern American,* 8(1): 5-17.

Peletz, M. (2006). Transgenderism and gender pluralism in Southeast Asia since early modern times. *Current Anthropology*, *47*(2), 309–340.

Rosenlee, L.-H. (2023, Spring). Gender in Confucian philosophy. In E. N. Zalta & U. Nodelman (Eds.), *The Stanford Encyclopedia of Philosophy*, https://plato.stanford.edu/archives/spr2023/entries/confucian-gender

### Socio-Emotional Relationship Therapy

ChenFeng, J., Kim, L., Knudson-Martin, C., & Wu, Y. (2016). Application of socio-emotional relationship therapy with couples of Asian heritage: Addressing issues of culture, gender, and power. *Family Process*, 56:558–573. doi: 10.1111/famp.12251

Knudson-Martin, C. (2023). *A step-by-step guide to socio-emotional relationship therapy: A socially responsible approach to clinical practice* (1st ed.). Routledge. https://doi.org/10.4324/9781003270232

Knudson-Martin, C., Wells, M., & Samman, S. (Eds.). (2015). *Socio-emotional relationship therapy: Bridging societal context, emotion, and power. Springer series in family therapy*. Springer.

# Part II

# Resistance, Resilience, and Imagined Possibilities

Counted out by eye shapes and last names
American bombs that made the earth shake, green cards, nail salons, and paper families
And they did it all in one take
Kids of immigrants
Who build our own ladders, duck snakes, upgraded from board game to board members
I'm so proud of my sister
No documents, now she writes her own chapters
No FAFSA but that paper in the mattress
Cash payments lookin funny on the taxes
Uncle Sam movin funny round the atlas
Consider it repayment for trauma of ancestors
I'm dancin wit my grandma at my cousin's weddin
Lookin at her, like your life is such a blessin
Matriarch, 94, still at the Y swimmin
Continue what she started, this is all just the beginnin

Jason Chu. (2023). Make it out [Song]. On *We Were the Seeds*. STILLONIT; KOEY Beats; Jonum.

DOI: 10.4324/9781003321590-6

# Part II

# Resistance, Resilience, and Imagined Possibilities

Chapter 4

# Beyond White Caricatures and Portrayals

## Asian American Therapists Shifting the Narrative

*Michael Chen*

The Yellow Peril was a term used in the late 19th century in the United States to describe the danger that the growing presence of Chinese immigrants posed to the white majority (Tsu, 2005). As Black slaves in America were emancipated, the country looked to other sources of labor to build its empire. As their numbers grew and cultural enclaves like Chinatown emerged, racist images and stereotypes published in newspapers (Fig. 4.1, 1899 editorial cartoon "The Yellow Terror in All His Glory") stoked fear, suspicion, and violence. And today, in the past several years, particularly in light of the COVID-19 pandemic and President Trump's *kung flu* remarks, a dramatic increase in overt anti-Asian hate has resurrected this sentiment in our country, raising mental health and public safety concerns for those of Asian descent (Liu et al., 2023).

On January 18, 2023, an Asian woman, 18 years old, was stabbed in the ear seven times by a white woman with a knife on a bus in Bloomington, Indiana. The woman was arrested and admitted that she targeted this young woman because she thought she was Chinese, and that there would be "one less person to blow up our country." More than simply one individual's mental illness, larger systemic forces have created and shaped narratives that impact the lived experiences of Asian Americans in the United States. This chapter examines how white supremacist portrayals of Asian Americans in media and societal discourse have shaped oppressive stereotypes that exist today, and how they shape the therapeutic process. The persistent and insidious nature of narratives targeting Asian Americans impacts the context of both Asian American therapists and clients alike. Where do these narratives come from? How are they being re-enacted today?

Michael White, a key figure in the development of narrative therapy, acknowledged that every human has meaning-making capacities and that the process of change was meant to elicit or re-activate these potentials toward unique outcomes (White, 2007). Narrative therapy is tied to post-modern philosophical frameworks which emphasize the deconstruction of dominant meta-narratives to prioritize individual agency within oppressive systems. This re-authoring process seeks to empower and liberate the client from old narratives—lived subconsciously—and a maladaptive identity that further entrenches problem-saturated

DOI: 10.4324/9781003321590-7

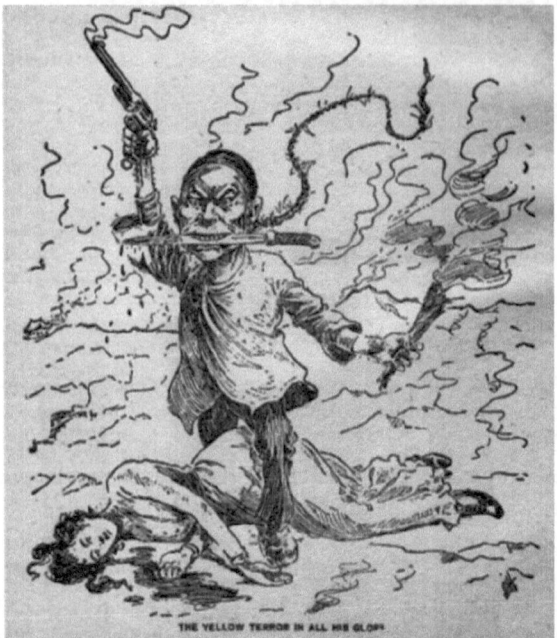

*Figure 4.1* "The Yellow Terror in All His Glory"

stories. John Bowlby (1988), pioneer of attachment theory, interviewed mothers who described traumatic childhoods but nonetheless raised children showing secure attachment. A characteristic of each of these mothers, who experienced post-traumatic growth, despite describing the experience of rejection and unhappiness during childhood, recounted positively that each was able to tell her story in a fluent and coherent way, in which positive aspects of their experiences were given due place and were integrated with all the negative ones (Bowlby, 1988). Thus, healing our stories through the framework of Narrative Therapy can address issues of collective and historical trauma for Asian Americans.

## Personal Narrative

As a second-generation Chinese American, my parents immigrated to the United States from Taiwan in 1965. Born amid bombing from Japan at the end of World War II, and facing impoverished conditions, they moved to America for further education, employment, and hopes of a better life. They ended up settling in the suburbs of St. Paul, Minnesota, after my father finished his PhD studies at the University of Minnesota. By all accounts, they had achieved the American dream by working, saving, and moving out of the city to a predominantly white suburb to raise their three young children.

Because of my parents' desire to remain in the United States to live in a context with white schools and white-bodied neighbors, the pressure to succeed by white cultural standards and conventions became an animating force for me. While my parents attempted to put me into Chinese language school on Saturdays, they also spoke English to me at home, reinforcing the narrative that assimilation would be the ultimate goal. Yet, fitting in was never a straightforward and simple reality, rather it entailed the loss of cultural expression, and fueled a deep internalized racism.

Starting at the age of five I realized that I did not belong—anywhere. A kindergarten classmate was sure to let me know that I was "yellow" and that he was white, and a trip to Taiwan to visit my parents' homeland was accompanied by mockery and humiliation for not speaking Mandarin. Indeed, the complexity of my family system is framed by migration trauma and the dissonance related to the immigrant experience experienced in my own body.

The pressure to assimilate, financial instability, language barriers, and lack of emotional support led to my parents' eventual divorce. Divorce is very uncommon in Asian families and considered shameful. In a conversation about their divorce and marital strife, I recall my dad explicitly instructing me, "Don't tell anyone about this." In the collective context that has historically emphasized honor and shame, I often felt like I had to hide and put on a good face. While outwardly successful, my interior experience was rife with turmoil and heartache. It wasn't safe to express sadness or grief in my family system, and to tell others would mean I would betray my family. Every day there was concern and material support—love was equated to material provision and labor—yet from a very early age I had to learn to navigate this uncertain and dangerous emotional landscape.

In Bowenian terms, I was cut off from my family story and cultural history. This growing sense of fragmentation led to loss of language, shame regarding my own name, and self-contempt for my own face. More than cognitive dissonance, this dislocation was felt and experienced in my body, and no matter how many compliments I received, and how many accolades and awards I won, the gnawing sense of living in-between two worlds led to a deep depression during high school. This darkness led to a slowing down, and a search for meaning, that ultimately led me on a path of healing and transformation that has taken decades. One of the key principles has been adopting the viewpoint of cultural somatics. As womanist scholars have noted, our *bodies* are the texts that carry the memories and pieces of the narrative (Cannon, 1993). Racism and the stereotypes about Asians are never abstract but center on the body, whether it is slanted eyes or flat faces, shame lands and lives in us through our embodied experiences.

Epigenetics is a field of study, pioneered by Rachel Yehuda, that examines the impact of intergenerational trauma on the person in specific historical and

cultural contexts. Yehuda examined both the psychological and physiologi-
cal impact of the Holocaust on subsequent generations of survivors and their
families (Yehuda & Bierer, 2009). Others have examined the impact of chattel
slavery on the psyche and the body of African descendants and their family
systems (Grossi, 2020). To strengthen the evidence further, a landmark epigenetic study done on mice demonstrated that trauma is passed on at the DNA
level in successive generations where high levels of hyper-vigilance and anxiety
were clearly noted in the offspring of traumatized mice (Dias & Ressler, 2014).
This positive finding makes very clear the connection between trauma and the
impact on the body. However, these data points led me to wonder, *what about
the Asian American story*? How has *my body* been carrying trauma? And on the
other hand, how does my body bear witness to the resilience and strength of my
people?

Because access to stories, collective memory, and tradition has been cut off
or greatly limited through migration for children of the diaspora, coupled with
the strong drive to assimilate, many Asian Americans are left to contend with
the stereotypes of Asian Americans as portrayed in television, film, and social
media. In 1869 the original photograph commemorating the completion of the
transcontinental railroad excluded the many Chinese laborers that had risked
their lives and provided countless hours working in dangerous conditions to
provide the infrastructure for commerce in this country (The Gilder Lehrman
Institute of American History, 2012). A story was being told about a people and
a place that did not give voice to the many thousands of Chinese immigrants and
did not honor their lived experiences. This was a pivotal moment in American
history that continues to be re-enacted through erasure and invisibility.

As a former campus minister at the University of Pennsylvania, mental health
came into sharp focus several years ago as a number of suicides on campus
occurred together within a short period. The suicide of a white woman on the
Penn Track and Field team garnered much attention, including spotlights on
ESPN and other national news media outlets, while the death of Asian students
remained obscured by the wishes of family to remain anonymous, and perhaps
avoid further shame and humiliation. While privacy in sensitive matters is a right
given to the families, at times complicating communication, it reveals the bind
of being seen and known, as an Asian American. This silence has the impact
of leaving our communities and stories unknown, unheard, misunderstood, and
inscrutable in the eyes of others.

## Asian Americans and the Body

There is inherent complexity in being seen as an Asian in America. The body,
for Asian Americans, is contested territory. It is a paradoxical body. To engage
in a therapeutic relationship as an Asian American is to acknowledge and engage

the ambivalence of being a body in a system that cannot bear the complexity of individuals and families—rendering them unassimilable. On the one hand Asians are both seen and needed for their labor and for their industriousness: Chinese and Filipino men and women, as early as the 16th century, left their homes to find themselves ensnared and coerced into dangerous systems where they bore the brunt of the rapacious desire to build the Western portion of the United States, making Asians highly useful. And on the other hand, as their numbers increased, fear and xenophobia gave way to systematic oppression through the passage of laws that excluded entrance into the country (Lee, 2016). These laws were not merely aimed at exclusion but in reality the extermination of the Chinese and those of Asian descent. The notion that Asians are both useful and dangerous has created a complex reality marked by economic demand, exploitation, and violence.

As a therapist, what images come to mind when you think about Asian Americans? Post World War II, and Japanese internment, sociologists began to see the survival of Japanese Americans as a success story. As immigration to the United States opened up in 1965 to educated and highly skilled laborers, Asian Americans were identified as a Model Minority in America (Eng & Han, 2019). This stereotype has been detrimental to overall health outcomes as it has heaped heavy burdens on Asian Americans to perform academically and vocationally while sacrificing their mental health. "Asian American" is an umbrella term that includes nearly 40 sub-groups, each with their own language, customs, and culture. Originally, student protestors in the 1970s coined the term Asian American as a unifying term for political action and advocacy. Today it is used as a demographic term, and in that there is a diminishment of nuances between people groups and loss of cultural particularity and ultimately, human dignity. Asian Americans have the largest intra-group wealth gap (Kochnar & Cilluffo, 2018); rates of poverty are high in Southeast Asian communities, and ostensibly these factors weigh heavily on health outcomes. Therapists need to take the time to dismantle and deconstruct their own personal biases and preconceived notions of what they have seen or heard in the news and media about Asian Americans.

## Beginnings and the Therapeutic Alliance

The Model Minority Myth has also had other deleterious effects. In the racial hierarchy in the United States, Asians are caught between Blacks and whites. Racial Triangulation (Xu & Lee, 2013) refers to the experience of many Asian Americans finding themselves caught in the tension of hierarchy, power, and representation in the United States. The model minority stereotype is a backhanded compliment that pushes Asians toward being honorary whites (Tuan, 1998), while at the same time stoking racial tension between Blacks and Asians; minority groups are pitted against one another in a game where everyone loses, and those in power remain "benevolent parents" to the quarreling siblings. Racial triangulation and the narratives that have emerged out of these experiences have provoked anger and self-contempt in the lives of Asian Americans, as well as the feeling of despair in being perpetual foreigners. In a therapeutic alliance, it may be critical to validate this particular experience, to name it as racial triangulation, and to make room for a multiplicity of stories to be told and honored, and to give permission to the full range of human emotion. Powerful emotions like anger need to be validated, particularly in the lives of Asian Americans who have learned to suppress anger and other strong emotions so as not to disturb the harmony in the family system, or even the racial hierarchy in the United States. Thus, for an Asian American in a therapeutic setting not to have to be the good boy or girl can be powerfully healing.

## Engaging Narratives of Race, Gender, and Power

Deconstructing deeply problematic narratives is part of the healing process for both individual and collective bodies. Negative appraisals and stereotypes are never abstractions but aimed at the lived experience of bodies in particular times and spaces. Historically, Asian women have been eroticized and are very often the object of sexual fetish as they are seen as clean and submissive. Asian men are seen as either nerdy and effeminate on one the hand or as terrorists and kung fu heroes on the other hand. These dehumanizing stereotypes are historical in nature yet have major implications for Asian Americans in the present day.

### Asian American Men and Emasculation

The historical context for Asian American men in particular is that of erasure and emasculation. The early wave of Chinese immigrants to the United States was met with discrimination and marginalization (Lee, 2016); primarily through exclusionary laws, they were forced into low-paying jobs that only women held, particularly, running laundromats. Anti-immigration laws also cut men off from their wives and families, which emasculated Asian men through cutting off a structure wherein they might demonstrate their strength and ability to offer provision and protection. Subsequently, anti-miscegenation laws also prohibited them from marrying outside of their race. These laws, in addition to daily discrimination, left Asian men contending with the narrative that they were both unwanted and undesirable—messages that they consistently face to this day.

Today, when it comes to dating and romantic relationships, Asian American men in particular are seen as very undesirable sexual partners. OKCupid published five years' worth of data from their app on race, gender, and attractiveness and showed that Asian men and Black women were consistently rated as "less attractive" than their same-gender counterparts (Kao, Balistreri, & Joyner, 2018). In fact, their study showed that white women rated Asian men 12% less attractive than average, and Asian women rated white men 16% more attractive than average. Thus, Asian men live within a tension of needing to be a model minority to succeed in the realms of academia and business—all indications point to Asian American men having higher than average income and educational attainment—yet they still find themselves less desirable sexually speaking.

Because of the negative appraisal of Asian men as sexual partners, body image issues present a challenge to their mental health. In a study on body issues in Asian men, participants expressed confusion over what an ideal masculine body type would be, and this confusion was directly tied to the ambivalence of fitting into the Western ideal of hegemonic masculinity (Liao et al., 2020). Bulking up through weight gain and obsessive working out may be an issue connected to the damaging narrative of the effeminate Asian man. And more specifically, small penis size has been a long-term stereotype that Asian men still contend with on a regular basis. The issue of emasculation for Asian American men is so pervasive that this experience extends into different spheres of life.

Members of the media feel emboldened to use this stereotype to harm, injure, and degrade. After NBA basketball player Jeremy Lin, a Taiwanese American man, exploded onto the scene in 2012 with a number of high-scoring games, reporter Jason Whitlock tweeted, "Some lucky lady in NYC is gonna feel a couple inches of pain tonight." The emasculation of both Asian American men and women in the United States has a long history, and the old narratives that Asian men are weak, effeminate, and pliable are still playing out today. Despite the individual global success of Filipino boxing star Manny Pacquiao, Arnaldo (2016) sees his masculinity in relationship to the Filipina/o community in America as both complicated and "falling short of liberatory potential" because of the larger social and economic forces at play in his popularity as well as the enduring narratives of the weak, effeminate, and savage body of the Filipino male.

One of the key reasons stereotypes of the nerdy and effeminate man persist is the lack of representation in television, film, and media of emotionally complex and sexually attractive leading Asian men. While there are examples of Asian men as either sexual or physical threats in film, there are so few examples of Asian men as romantic leads in movies. Because of this void, the narrative of the unfeeling, robotic, and nerdy man remains lodged in the collective consciousness. Steven Yeun, who played Glenn on the television show "The Walking Dead" is one of the few examples in recent history of an Asian man getting the girl—a white woman no less! Despite the fact that he has low self-esteem, starting the show off as a pizza delivery boy, and has to be convinced by the female protagonist of the show that he is both a worthy romantic partner and good leader, it continues to serve as inspiration and validation to many Asian men. To this day, Yeun is still receiving emails from fans of the show who applaud him for his portrayal of Glenn (Kang, 2021), one that raised the romantic prospects and sexual appraisal of Asian men in America.

### Asian American Women Fetishization and Violence

The narratives about Asian American women also persist. The earliest accounts of Asian female bodies coming to North America via the trans Pacific slave trade created the context for exploitation and violence done to Asian women. Mirrha Catarina is one of the earliest and paradigmatic stories we have of an Asian female in the Americas (Myers, 2003). Her exact birthplace is unknown, but was of South Asian descent. As a girl, she was kidnapped by Portuguese slavers and ended up in Manila to be sold to a high-ranking official in Mexico, presumably to be used as a sex worker or concubine. Providentially, she ends up in the family of devout Catholics who rename her Mirrha-Catarina. It is thought she continues to wear her Indian sari or keeps some vestige of it, while adopting traditional Mexican clothing. The style is now known as *China Poblana* (Fig. 4.2, the China Poblana style blouse and skirt)—a symbol of a woman that is both a clean, submissive servant and yet too sexually promiscuous. Her Indian roots are erased as she becomes venerated as the ideal Mexican woman, and her

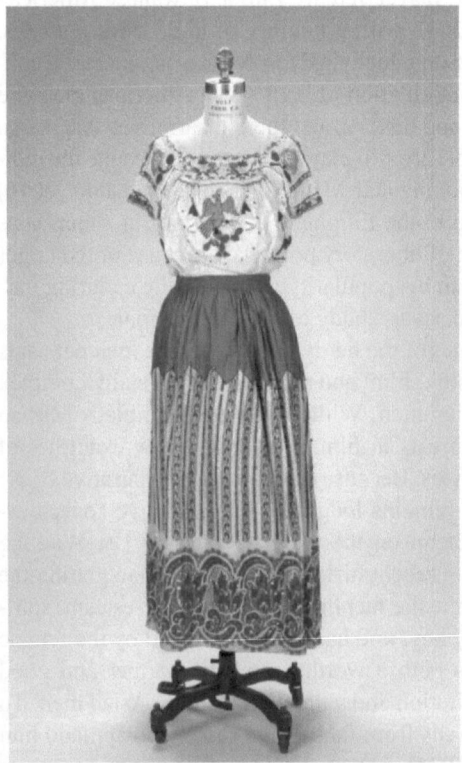

*Figure 4.2* China poblana

story is written, interpreted, and banned through religious and colonial lenses (Gillespie, 1998)

Asian immigrant women have endured a long history of sexual victimization in the United States. Chinese women in the 1840s were commonly seen as filthy, void of domestic value, lustful, and sensual. These women, lured into relocating to the United States in promise of a better life, were often subject to racial discrimination and forced into prostitution. By 1860, over 23.4 percent of Chinese (all women) in San Francisco were employed in commercial sex and prostitution (Almaguer, 1994). Damaging narratives have led to sexual exploitation that persists even today. According to a 2016 study, 4.8 million people were forced into sexual slavery globally; and seven out of ten were women from the Asia and Pacific region (International Labor Office, 2017). And even as recent as 2021, six women of Asian descent were killed while working at a spa in Atlanta. The perpetrator, a young white male, insisted that he killed these women because they were a sexual temptation to him. Without knowing the long history of hyper-sexualization of Asian women reinforced through economic systems, one might be led to see these deaths as isolated incidents rather than part of the deep sickness of this country.

## Trauma, Resilience, and New Narratives

Powerful connections can be made to trauma studies and narrative structure. It is well documented that normal memory and traumatic memory differ greatly (Van Der Kolk, 2014). Normal memory is sorted into coherent narrative forms that are somewhat flexible, while traumatic memory is rigid and frightful and lacks a sense of time and context. Trauma brings fragmentation, wherein the meaning-making parts of our brain go off-line, and the construction of a coherent narrative—one with beginning, middle, and end—is impossible (Van Der Kolk, 2014). To be human is to wrestle with the impact of trauma and its devastating impact on our ability to construct coherent narrative in both an individual and collective sense. Out of this pain, individuals seek relief through addiction and various coping mechanisms or fall into melancholy or dissociation. Absent a strong sense of narrative, perpetrators re-enact violence rooted in harmful narratives that are perpetuated through mass media. Thus, when self-determination occurs through narrative means, there must be an acknowledgment of the dehumanizing stereotypes that prevail in our context and also must entail a search to construct new stories with new possibilities. As Asian Americans, if we are not writing our own stories, someone else will be writing and interpreting them for us.

Collective trauma speaks to the reality that not only do individuals suffer abuse, neglect, and great harm, but that entire people groups face genocide, holocaust, and oppression that affects multiple generations. Rea Tajiri is the daughter of survivors of Japanese internment. In the fragmentation, loss of memory, and her parents' inability to construct the narrative, she created a documentary regarding her search for history and identity to fill an aching void and to address the feelings she had of being unmoored like a ghost floating over water. Tajiri (1991) states, "For years, I've been living with this picture without the story, feeling a lot of pain, not knowing how they fit together." The ability to know how events from the past shape our present and our future is what it means to become human.

Because Asian American stories have consistently been erased or marginalized, many stories have gone untold, leaving history to repeat itself. There is currently no museum or experience that tells a comprehensive story of Asian American history, trauma, and resilience. Without these stories being told, the loss of language, traditions, and culture impacts both families and individuals and their sense of cohesion and identity, making Asian Americans vulnerable to the violence of capitalist systems. Obsession with the productive Asian body brought thousands to the United States, fear and contempt of these same bodies tore them apart in Los Angeles during the Chinese Massacre of 1871. A violent mob stormed Chinatown which led to the lynching of 21 Chinese men—the largest mass lynching in U.S. history (Lee, 2016).

## Learning the Past, Shaping the Future

Subsequently, Angel Island near San Francisco was the initial point of entry for many Chinese in the early 1900s. It was the parallel experience to Ellis Island on the East Coast for many European immigrants. While the white immigrants at Ellis Island breezed through customs, the Chinese were detained for months at Angel Island, stripped naked, humiliated, and forced into barracks—these were truly strangers from a different shore (Takaki, 1989). Within these barracks, hundreds of poems carved into the walls in Chinese calligraphy were discovered 30 years later, some under many layers of paint, expressing a deep anguish over the unjust and harsh treatment upon entering the country. In a sense, these poems can be considered the first Asian American literature and reveal the nature of power, protest, and narrative in our own words. The discovery of the past revealed untold stories that began the healing process for many and have subsequently inspired works of art, music, and collective action.

In light of persistent exclusion and erasure, anti-Asian hate cannot be simply confined to individual transgression but must be seen in light of larger systemic forces. Asian immigrants since their arrival to the United States have faced discrimination and violence based on their race, and thus, these cannot merely be isolated incidents or someone's personal moral shortcomings or even simply the mental illness of individuals, but it is collective in nature and has corporate implications. For centuries now the Asian American community has been wrestling with how to make sense of trauma in narrative form. Is there hope for us as a people living in the midst of systems of exploitation and violence? What examples of resilience within the Asian American community can we identify as creative narrative work that engages collective trauma?

One source and protective factor over many years for Asians coming to the United States for the first time has been the church—a source for corporate gathering and meaning-making. While Asian Americans identify with a wide array of religions and spiritual practices, Christian churches have not only provided hope in a liturgical and spiritual sense but have also played a critical role in community support and even providing material needs for those new to the country. The Asian American church has in some cases assimilated into white church systems and denominations, while others have wrestled with the meta-narrative of trauma, existence, in their own cultural meaning-making process. The long-standing exclusion and oppression of Asian Americans led Korean Christian theologians to discuss the concept of *han*, as Yoo (1988) explains, it is the

> feeling of unresolved resentment against injustices suffered, a sense of helplessness because of the overwhelming odds against one, a feeling of acute pain in one's guts and bowels, making the whole body writhe and squirm, and an obstinate urge to take revenge and to right the wrong—all these combined.
>
> (p. 221)

Christ, in this theological paradigm, is the one who must resolve the feeling and experience of *han*. Related to this is *minjung* theology, in which Jesus is conceptualized as a shamanistic priest whose blood has power to heal. I would contend that to grow and heal as Asian Americans we need to continue to process the meaning and importance of our cultural past, including both material and spiritual resources, as it pertains to hope for our future. The following case study seeks to illustrate the inextricable link between collective and individual narratives playing out in the therapeutic process.

### Case of Allan

Allan, age 35, a second-generation Chinese American male, began therapy reporting mild depression. Single and without children, he is generally well-liked at his job as he works for a marketing company in New York City. Born in the United States, in a predominantly white suburb, Allan moved to New York City to attend New York University and has lived there since college. Below is a portion of a therapy session with Allan where he begins to engage with the harm done to him that he has not yet processed, which subsequently remains enigmatic.

*ALLAN:* I am not sure why, but I feel depressed…a real lack of motivation, and at the same time I feel really angry, a rage that I don't like. I don't like that about myself… I often feel annoyed and easily irritated.

*THERAPIST:* Is that everywhere? At home? Or at work?

*ALLAN:* Yeah, pretty much everywhere. At work, my boss hired this new guy, some hot shot in marketing, and started to just give him a lot of control over different areas, different projects. For a while this guy is complimenting me on my hair, my style, whatever, then in our first in person meeting, while we're in line waiting for lunch, he jabs his finger up into my ass.

*THERAPIST:* [nodding] Hmm. [concerned]

*ALLAN:* Like what the fuck man? I was pissed, and then just had to eat it, like I have to work with this guy, so I just stuff it down. It was like a game to him, a locker room thing...

*THERAPIST:* Hm. That's really awful. I'm sorry that happened to you. White guy?

*ALLAN:* Yeah, white guy. And now, I am just making the connection, like this is not the first time that happened to me...When I was 15 years old, I was in a high school musical and the lead of the play, during a rehearsal, jammed his finger up into my rectal area. I mean we were weeks into rehearsals, going over the moves for a scene with Nathan and the guys. We were in several rows. Hands up, hands down. Hands up, hands down. Side step, side step. I was working hard to remember all these steps and in order—when I felt up into my rectum, a finger jammed and wriggled hard. It was Andy Ferkus, I looked back out of my peripheral vision, and heard his mocking laughter. The director didn't see anything but me out of sync in the rehearsal. I was pissed then too, and just stuffed all that emotion down, way down. What was I supposed to do, tell the director the star of the theater department rammed his finger up into my ass, please tell him to stop it?

*THERAPIST:* No, it's terrible. And you've never told anyone?

*ALLAN:* No. Like I said, I just take and feel like I can't say anything.

*THERAPIST:* What do you make of the fact that the *same thing* happened to you, some 20 years apart?

*ALLAN:* [despondent] I don't know...it just doesn't make any sense to me.

*THERAPIST:* Do you think it's connected to your depression?

*ALLAN:* Yeah, maybe. I was *really* depressed in high school.

Over the course of several months, tremendous feelings of anger are eventually met with grief, as the experience in his body of feeling unwelcome—the perpetual foreigner—in every space started to emerge. Years of bottling up the grief and anger led to somatic issues: chronic migraines, indigestion, and insomnia. These slowly began to resolve over the course of therapy.

While Allan was well-liked as a person in most cases, we began to connect his experience of violence to the historical narrative of the effeminate Chinese man. The fact that he will always be in a position of submission without recourse—*perfect* for middle management—and that is the lot for Asian men. This starts to settle in for Allan.

One of the most notable features of the healing process for Allan was the feeling of relief in knowing that he was not alone in his experiences as an Asian man. Learning about the long history of the emasculation of Chinese men in this country gave a frame of reference to understand his own trauma. The re-enactment of the assault on his body, and his dignity, was essentially a recapitulation of violence done to Asian men in the United States beginning in the 1800s, a subconscious re-enactment rendering the Asian male body both desired and useful, and yet made vulnerable to violence.

We discussed Marco Polo's legendary tales of the orient, how it inspired Christopher Columbus to search after the wealth and splendor of Indians in South Asia so that it might be plundered. The rapacious desire to conquer and consume led to violence against Indigenous bodies, Columbus mistaking Native Americans for South Asians, all with the *orientalist narrative* that there are riches in the Asian collective body to be used and plundered. For Allan, his depression gave way to indignation and disbelief as he came to realize that the same narrative about Asian culture and bodies was playing out in his own experience; it wasn't a distant culture or far-away point in history, but rather it was his body that became the object of exploitation and degradation.

## Conclusion

The field of Marriage and Family Therapy has largely been pioneered by white bodies with little attention to issues pertaining to Asian Americans, and diversity in higher educational systems can easily fall into a Black and white binary. In light of the absence of Asian Americans in the field advancing systemic thought through clinical practice and scholarship, where are we to turn? One of the dehumanizing stereotypes that Asians continually deal with is that we are quiet, cold, robotic, and unfeeling. Narrative healing then has meant re-discovering emotionally complex resources for healing within ancient thought.

Recovering and reclaiming ancient symbols, rituals, and philosophy is part of the narrative work we have in seeing ourselves as part of a larger story—a story that is even longer than our recent memory of immigration. We are not alone. We have not been cut off, but bear in our bodies the collective wisdom and practice of those who have come before us. One of the key symbols in ancient Chinese thought is the circle containing dual and oppositional forces known as the *yinyang* symbol.

The *yinyang* symbol is shorthand for a larger system of thought. Philosopher and writer Zhou Danyi emerged from a noble family in the Song Dynasty of the 11th century and became one of the most important figures in a Neo-Confucianist movement of scholars and practitioners. He sought to bridge the ethics of Confucius with the philosophy of Daoism (Wang, 2005).

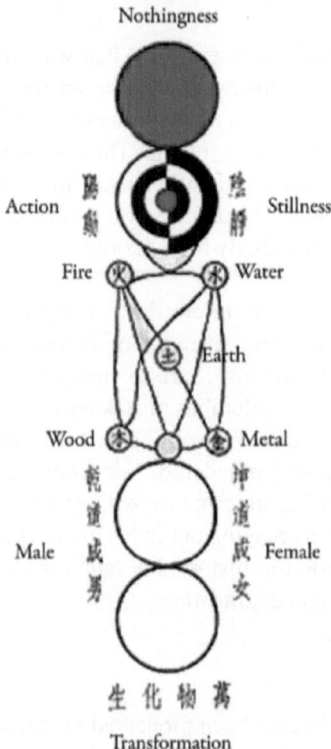

*Figure 4.3* Taijitu Shuo

Zhou's philosophical system—a cosmology of creative energy—begins with the supreme ultimate (Nothingness) but is deeply intertwined with nature and human systems. Figure 4.3 (*Taijitu of Zhou Danyi*) shows from top to bottom the creative energy and transformation emerging from the interplay of oppositional forces. From the beginning, the supreme ultimate moves and generates *yang* (masculine, active, positive energy) which generates rest and *yin* (feminine, still-ness, negative energy). The presence and movement of these forces yield the five elements: wood, fire, air, water, and metal. In turn these elements diffuse harmoniously and give rise to seasons. Male and female emerge out of heaven and earth, and the energy of these two leads to boundless changes and infinite transformations.

Where does this cosmology lead? Self-cultivation is the notion of develop-ment, refinement, and growth in wisdom. Zhou insists that the sage is the one who seeks harmony and balance and embraces the mutuality of opposing forces, and in so doing becomes as bright as the stars in the heavens. In particular, it is in learning to harmonize righteousness and benevolence that one becomes truly established as a sage.

Rather than prescribing a technique or methodology for wellness, Zhou provides an eco-systemic lens as a theory of change that connects creation, nature, and emotional regulation. Thus to grow in one's capacity to bear in the body oppositional forces: the tension of light and darkness, masculine and feminine, strength and tenderness. This is what it means to become a truly wise person, living out benevolence, righteousness, propriety, wisdom, and trust in relationships and human affairs to produce the state of tranquility and rest.

Moreover, it is in harmonizing the polarity of righteousness (strength) and benevolence (tenderness) that one becomes a sage. Wang (2005) translates Zhou's central thought in learning to both embrace and balance these seemingly oppositional forces to become a sage:

> In nature, there are hardness and softness (which may result in) goodness or evil. All (is right) when there is the mean (*zhong*). (This explanation) not being understood, (Zhou) continued: The goodness that results from hardness consists of righteousness (*yi*), straightforwardness (*chih*), decisiveness, strictness, firmness, determination, and steadfastness. The evil resulting from it consists of ruthlessness, intolerance, force, and violence. The goodness that results from softness consists of compliance and docility. The evil resulting from it consists of weakness of will, indecisiveness, and underhanded sycophancy. The mean (*zhong*) signifies harmony and proper proportion. This alone is the highest Way (*Tao*) of the world and the concern of the sage. Hence the sage emphasizes those teachings which will cause men to reform their evils of themselves, proceed by themselves to the mean, and there stop.
>
> (p. 319)

There is simplicity, brilliance, mystery, and paradox in the acknowledgment that we contend with ambivalence on a daily basis in nearly every area of life. Ambivalence is a good thing and part of the creative process of becoming more authentically human. In discovering Zhou, I realized that I am not alone as an Asian man in the field of Marriage and Family Therapy, and that I come from a long line of healers, sages, and prophets. I am no longer threatened by the notion of the emasculated Asian male body—because I can embrace feminine/masculine energy—and I bless my anger as an integral part of the unity of righteousness/benevolence, and find that harmonizing these energies has potential to create space for others to find sanctuary within themselves.

Asian Americans bring many strengths and unique perspectives to the therapeutic process—priorities in collective consciousness that have emerged over many centuries passed down to us as resilience through our bodies enacted in the rituals of family meals and celebrations. And as the demographic reality of

Asian Americans continues to evolve, what we bring is a present unfolding, something dynamic and *in-process* as we ponder who we are. What does it mean to bring your whole self to the therapeutic process for me as an Asian American man with Taiwanese heritage? It is to live with paradox in an embodied sense that the one is many, and the many are one. I bring the voices of my people, and there is ancient wisdom that lives in my bones that can bring healing to both individual clients and to communities. I conclude with a poem written to address the person of the therapist in long narrative perspective of what I bring to each and every therapeutic engagement:

> I am never alone.
> I bring a whole village.
> Of prophets, poets, warriors, and sages
> Rich in language, philosophy
> I also bring tea pots of welcome
> brimming with the oolong tea of the High Mountains in the Hsinchu province
> The ground of my father's birth
> It is in my body, and there is always enough
> wisdom to be shared, knowledge to enrich,
> And honor to bestow

## Reflection Questions

### Questions for the Therapist

1.  As a therapist, what images come to mind when you think about Asian Americans? From your earliest experiences, what has shaped your perception and imagination for the lives of Asian Americans?
2.  Asian Americans often see themselves as caught between unresolvable tensions, how does this chapter help your understanding of working through liminal spaces? What is your own relationship to ambivalence and how do you resolve the binds you find yourself in?
3.  In this chapter, the author makes the case that reclaiming one's cultural past is integral to healing work. Do you agree? What might that look like for you and your clients?
4.  Where might you need to continue to process your cultural heritage and the impact on your *body* as the text that carries the story in your position as a therapist?

### Questions for Therapy

1.  Where do you see racial re-enactments happening today in your context, and what is the impact on you and your community?

2. In this chapter one example of shifting the narrative was provided for Asian Americans, what other ways might you participate in deconstructing harmful narratives in the lives of clients?

3. Where might you need to continue to process your cultural heritage and the impact on your *body* as the text that carries the story?

## References

Almaguer, T. (1994). *Racial fault lines: The historical origins of white supremacy in California.* University of California Press.

Arnaldo, C. (2016). "I'm Thankful for Manny": Manny Pacquiao, Pugilistic Nationalism, and the Filipina/o Body. In S. Davé, L. Nishime, & T. Oren (Eds.), *Global Asian American popular cultures* (pp. 27–45). New York University Press.

Bowlby, J. (1988). *A secure base: Parent-child attachment and healthy human development.* Basic Books.

Cannon, K. G. (1993). Womanist perspectival discourse and cannon formation. *Journal of Feminist Studies in Religion, 9*(1/2), 29–37. www.jstor.org/stable/25002198

Dias, B., & Ressler, K. (2014). Parental olfactory experience influences behavior and neural structure in subsequent generations. *Nature Neuroscience 17*, 89–96. https://doi.org/10.1038/nn.3594

Eng, D., & Han, S. (2019). *Racial melancholia, racial dissociation: On the social and psychic lives of Asian Americans.* Duke University Press. https://doi.org/10.1215/9781478002680

The Gilder Lehrman Institute of American History. (2012). *Official photograph from the "Golden Spike" Ceremony, 1869.* https://www.gilderlehrman.org/history-resources/spotlight-primary-source/official-photograph-golden-spike-ceremony-1869

Gillespie, J. L. (1998). Gender, ethnicity and piety: The case of the *China Poblana.* In Bueno & Caesar (Eds.), *Imagination beyond nation: Latin American popular culture* (pp. 19–37). University of Pittsburgh Press.

Grossi, É. (2020). New avenues in epigenetic research about race: Online activism around reparations for slavery in the United States. *Social Science Information, 59*(1), 93–116. https://doi.org/10.1177/0539018419899336

International Labor Office. (2017). *Global estimates of modern slavery: Forced labour and forced marriage.* ILO Publications.

Kang, J. C. (2021, February 7). The many lives of Steven Yeun. *The New York Times Magazine, 24.*

Kao, G., Balistreri, K. S., & Joyner, K. (2018). Asian American men in romantic dating markets. *Contexts, 17*(4), 48–53. https://doi.org/10.1177/1536504218812869

Kochnar, R. and Cilluffo, A. (2018). Income inequality in the U.S. is rising most rapidly among Asians. Pew Research Center. https://www.pewsocialtrends.org/2018/07/12/income-inequality-in-the-u-s-is-rising-most-rapidly-among-asians/

Lee, E. (2016). *The making of Asian America: A history.* Simon & Schuster.

Liao, K. Y., Shen, F. C., Cox, A. R., Miller, A. R., Sievers, B., & Werner, B. (2020). Asian American men's body image concerns: A focus group study. *Psychology of Men & Masculinity, 21*(3), 333–344. https://doi.org/10.1037/men0000234

Liu, M., Anastasio, N., LeFreniere, H., & Perliger, A. (2023). Public health crisis and hate crimes: Deciphering the proliferation of Anti-Asian violence in the US before and during COVID-19. *Perspectives on Terrorism*, 17(2), 30–59. https://www.jstor.org/stable/27255591

Myers, K. A. (2003). *Neither saints nor sinners: Writing the lives of women in Spanish America*. Oxford University Press. https://doi.org/10.1093/acprof:oso/9780195157239.001.0001

Tajiri, R. (1991). *History and memory: For Akiko and Takashige* [Film]. Women Make Movies.

Takaki, R. T. (1989). *Strangers from a different shore: A history of Asian Americans*. Little, Brown.

Tsu, J. (2005). *Failure, nationalism, and literature: The making of modern Chinese identity, 1895–1937*. Stanford University Press.

Tuan, M. (1998). *Forever foreigners or honorary whites?: The Asian ethnic experience today*. Rutgers University Press.

Van der Kolk, B. A. (2014). *The body keeps the score: Brain, mind, and body in the healing of trauma*. Viking Press.

Wang, R. R. (2005). Zhou Dunyi's diagram of the Supreme Ultimate explained ("Taijitu shuo"): A construction of the confucian metaphysics. *Journal of the History of Ideas*, 66(3), 307–323. http://www.jstor.org/stable/3654184

White, M. (2007). *Maps of narrative practice*. W.W. Norton & Company.

Xu, J., & Lee, J. C. (2013). The marginalized "Model" minority: An empirical examination of the racial triangulation of Asian Americans. *Social Forces*, 91(4), 1363–1397.

Yehuda, R., & Bierer, L. M. (2009). The relevance of epigenetics to PTSD: Implications for the DSM-V. *Journal of Traumatic Stress*, 22(5), 427–434.

Yoo, B. (1988) *Korean pentecostalism: Its history and theology*. Verlag Peter Lang.

# Chapter 5

# Surviving Racism Across the Generations

## Quiet Fortitude to Active Resistance and Collective Healing

*Lana Kim and Jessica ChenFeng*

There are many vulnerabilities that come with existing in the U.S. as a person outside of the white majority. As Asian Americans, we know this well because we face racialized stress daily in both conscious and unconscious ways. From our everyday vigilance to avoid or deflect racist encounters, to managing down-played microaggressions, or the baseline stress we carry in bodies that are fet-ishized and considered forever foreign (Tuan, 1998), there is a psychological, emotional, and physical load we bear to live and be in this country. However, everyone does not experience, navigate, and manage racialized stress in the same way. How we do this relates to where we are with regard to time in history, loca-tion, the sociopolitical landscape, as well as our individual contexts, generation, and migration status. Our discussion about who we are in this country needs to include greater attention to the layers of context and how this shapes the realities of our lives. This chapter speaks to Asian American racism across the genera-tions, including the diversity seen within struggle and survival, and the genera-tive possibilities for carrying the legacy of resilience intentionally forward.

### Personal Connection to the Topic

This chapter is written from the perspectives of two, second-generation Asian American cisgender women, LK (Korean-Canadian) and JCF (Taiwanese-American) who were born to first-generation immigrants having differing migra-tion stories and economic backgrounds.

I (LK) was born and raised in Canada and came to the U.S. alone, in my mid-20s, to pursue graduate school. I have lived here now for almost 20 years. Living in the U.S., people assume that I am Asian American, and indeed, my Asian Canadian upbringing feels adjacent in many ways. However, my understanding of racism comes from witnessing and experiencing it through two different con-texts, Canada and the U.S., and the contrasting histories, sociopolitical contexts, and cultures of these countries. I grew up as the middle child and only daughter of first-generation immigrants from South Korea. My family's migration legacy

DOI: 10.4324/9781003321590-8

started with my father who came to Canada in 1970 during his early 20s through sponsorship by a white Canadian farming couple who had provided financial support for his education and housing as a child when he was left orphaned and with a physical disability from the Korean War. These people were his *parents* and my *Foremost grandparents (a small farming town in southern Alberta)*, as my brothers and I referred to them. My mother immigrated to Canada in the mid-1970s via marriage to my father when she was in her mid-20s.

My parents came to Canada with limited English skills, no higher education, and no marketable credentials, while also carrying powerful effects from the realities of the Korean War and its aftermath. On the other hand, they also brought with them determination, hope, and grit. They had survived unimaginable devastation in their country and their survival orientation was strong. My parents worked long hours, six days a week, in entry level service jobs until they started running their own small businesses where they did physically demanding work, the last being a dry cleaning shop they operated until their retirement. Despite their ceaseless efforts, their lives were characterized by financial hardship, and my brothers and I grew up helping my parents at work learning and living the immigrant struggle. They sacrificed much in order to provide opportunities and a better future for their children and I hold a consciousness about the privileges I hold because of this. Being second-generation, my native English fluency, educational status, professional status, and capital in its various forms is a felt, marked difference from the realities my first-generation parents lived.

My (JCF) parents were both born in Southern Taiwan, and the only lives they knew on the island nation were ones lived under martial law. It is a strange thing for me now to be learning about the sociopolitical history of Taiwan and experiencing some degree of cognitive dissonance – because my parents grew up in a Taiwan where there were consequences (including arrest, abduction or death) for talking about communist politics, writing simplified Chinese, or supporting Taiwan's independence. Mandarin Chinese was the only formal language in Taiwan and Tâi-oân-ōe/台灣話 (literally, "Taiwan language") was discouraged in school. These realities were not explicitly shared with us such that it gave shape to our understanding of being "from Taiwan." These reflections are my own sense-making of my parents' experiences.

My mother, the eldest of four daughters, was a teenager when her family felt the push to leave Taiwan due to the threat of Chinese communism. Like others who left Taiwan, their family first went to Buenos Aires, Argentina, leaving behind a fairly comfortable life (one that most likely, my grandparents shaped to shield their daughters from sociopolitical realities). My mother's dreams of becoming a physician were interrupted by being uprooted and having to finish high school in a new country with a new language. I marvel at her being able to fluently speak four languages now, finishing college in the U.S. and all the sacrifices she made as a young woman in order to give her own two daughters the life she dreamed of.

My father was the youngest of seven children and their family lived a modest life through the Japanese occupation and into the era of martial law. He has shared stories of our *ahma*/grandma having to make ends meet by hosting and feeding students and laborers in their home. My father followed his older siblings to the U.S.; though they all came for college and graduate studies (again, one way Asian migration was permitted due to the Hart-Celler Act), my father paved his own way through a life of being an entrepreneur. I remember the white colleagues and employees he had over the years and though he was their employer, I can still feel what I internalized from his experience as a sense of wanting to fit in, to be liked and accepted. The dream of being his own boss, though there were seasons this shaped economic privilege in our family's life, came with a lot of relational and contextual costs.

In our family system, I grew up with a lot of implicit responsibilities as the older daughter, caring for our parents' emotional well-being, reducing their stress by being "good," and making sure things were okay when my dad was out of the country for business trips. I have had the privilege to process through a lot of these experiences and in reflecting now, I finally have words to articulate some of these sentiments: that I have such a deep respect and gratitude for my parents' individual and collective capacities to endure through migration, profound personal loss/grief, and still envision a future of hope for their children and grandchildren. Their journeys are different from my own, and in appreciating the depth of their experiences, I can contextualize the journey my family is in this season and continue to dream as they have, for what our future can be.

## Immigrant Generation and Racialized Minority Stress

There is tremendous intra- and inter-group diversity among Asian Americans in the U.S., with foreign and U.S. born members across all age groups. Migration status and the context surrounding how and when migration happens also vary across time for different Asian ethnic groups. For example, the Pew Research Center states that the majority of Japanese Americans today are persons born in the U.S. since this ethnic group began arriving in Hawaii in the 19th century as plantation workers. In contrast, most Bhutanese Americans are currently first-generation immigrants who came to the U.S. more recently as refugees (Budiman & Ruiz, 2021). Therefore, while some Asian Americans are part of a generation that migrated, many others of us are U.S. born, yet the dominant assumption prevails that all Asians are immigrants (Lee, 2015).

The second-generation can include children born in the U.S. to more recent immigrants as well as adults like us who were born in the U.S. or other western countries such as Canada, to immigrants who arrived soon after the 1965 immigration reform. As second-generation Asian Americans who relate to the latter, we have often wondered how the minority stress we carry compares to what our first-generation immigrant parents endured and still face today. While we share phenotypic similarities, our versions of Asian America are distinctly different. We speak native English, the type of English that passes as "American" for its lack of Asian accent, and the way that we navigate societal systems and social contexts highlights our fluency with U.S. cultural norms. The first-generation had to assimilate, but being born in the U.S. we know how to speak the part, look the part, and socialize in a way that gains us a certain level of acceptance and membership, which more importantly, offers some protection from discrimination. This cultural capital is commonly taken for granted by those privileged to have it, but if you are located on the margins, you easily see the consequences for not being versed in mainstream culture and the ways this sets you back.

Though we are both second-generation Asians in North America, we know (from history, research, and lived experience) that third, fourth+ generation Asian Americans feel invisible because of this discourse and assumption that "all Asians are immigrants," leaving out the generations that these families have struggled through to establish a home in the U.S. Despite generational diversity among Asian Americans, being far removed from the immigrant generation does not automatically spare one from Asian American racialization which affects all who fit the phenotype.

## Their Struggle, Our Struggle

We know that in addition to minoritized racial identity and low levels of cultural capital, socioeconomic class (SES) is another major determinant of societal marginalization in the U.S. SES is arguably among the most influential factors that mediate societal power and privilege for immigrant groups. The SES class backgrounds of post-1965 first-generation Asian immigrants varied, but because the Immigration and Nationality Act (Hart-Celler Act) was designed to only allow highly skilled immigrants, many from this generation came well educated with advanced degrees and credentials from their countries of origin or to seek educational opportunities (Zhou & Kim, 2006). Therefore, some of us have parents wherein moving to the U.S. led to upward mobility, but this was not done without considerable struggle. One of the harsh realities common to the post-1965 first-generation immigrant experience was discrimination for accented English or lack of fluency and lingering anti-Asian sentiment which kept them from getting jobs in their fields (McClain, 1994). The result was financial instability and fighting through poverty and post-migration oppression, in the pursuit of a better life for their families.

Many second-generation Asian Americans similar to us know what it feels like as children to watch our parents with lower social capital and broken English navigate life in the U.S. with constant reminders of being on society's margins (Kim et al, 2019). The odds were stacked against them as they worked under stressful conditions to support their families and pursue some semblance of the

American dream that was not designed to include them. On some level, it is as if the downward mobility that often accompanies immigrant life was kind of an implicit social contract for the permission to live in this country. Many of us know first-hand that whether one came with skilled backgrounds, opportunities for the first-generation were often limited and relegated to menial jobs, manual labor such as janitorial or entry level factory line work, or creating small family businesses such as convenience stores, mom and pop restaurants, and laundromats. Already looked down upon because of race, accent, and foreignness, they were also disrespected by virtue of the work they had to do in order to survive in this land.

Whether our parents did blue- or white-collar work, they experienced the struggle of doing so from their marginalized status as first-generation immigrants. They survived in a time of the U.S. that held strongly to its long legacy of systemic racism and anti-Asian sentiment. The witnessing we as the second generation did was not only from a passive outsider position. It also impacted us and the family dynamics in our mixed migration status families. Some of these dynamics in immigrant families are related to the structural shifts in relational roles, and some of us may remember needing to intervene for our parents from early on as they had to rely on us to defend, translate, or broker their everyday situations with the white world. These roles and dynamics may still even persist today. The previous generation's struggle was also implicitly our struggle, and we internalized their pain. The vulnerability of witnessing our parents' vulnerability was visceral as we saw them experience overt and covert discrimination, judgment, and ridicule. The tension, stress, and mixed feelings of respect, appreciation, embarrassment, anger, and worry around these everyday experiences are ones many of us know well.

## Rebranding Anti-Asian Hate

Discrimination and xenophobia that the first generation endured are a key aspect of the vulnerability they faced. The anti-Asian hate shown today portrays racist actions, particularly physical and violent threats that are randomly committed in open, public spaces. These types of portrayals incite anxiety and fear regarding one's physical and psychological safety. They suggest a resurgence of racism toward Asian Americans and a rekindling of Yellow Peril sentiments (Li & Nicholson Jr., 2021). While the incidences of violence and assault publicized today are traumatic and bold, aggression and violence toward Asian Americans is not a new reality, but made to appear that way because of increased media coverage and attention where previously there was little interest. This rebranded form of racism obscures the type that has always existed and is actively enacted toward Asian American communities and alive in their consciousness (Gover et al., 2020). It needs to be named that Asians have endured and survived through centuries of anti-Asian hate in the U.S. (i.e., Chinese massacre of 1871, forced internment of Japanese Americans during World War II, attacks on South Asians based on phenotypic appearance following 9/11). There is also the long-standing prejudice that may not attack our bodies but is aimed at our psyche. We endure slurs muttered under one's breath, disgusted looks from passing drivers, annoyed glances in situations where one has innocently and unknowingly committed a social faux pas, job applications overlooked for less than perfect English, and sneers or racist jokes.

Anti-Asian hate is also perpetuated through societal attitudes that denigrate and other. Until more recently, anything representing *Asianness* was viewed as un-American and *less than,* which fuels ongoing marginalization. Whereas the model minority myth intentionally presents a skewed portrayal of Asian Americans as thriving against the odds, another side of the story is the theme of Asians as targets of humiliation. We know how it feels to internalize societally based shame around our heritage culture and identities that make us appear un-American. For example, one of my (LK) formative experiences around othering happened, like for many, during lunch at school. I remember the visceral embarrassment of being a fifth grader at school and my white peers, including my friends, darting disgusted looks or remarking "ew" in reaction to the smell of the kimbap my mom had woken up extra early to lovingly make. The shameful message sent was that Korean food was "gross" food. At that formative age, I took in the idea that *my* food was stinky and strange. Similarly, I developed a self-consciousness around other parts of my Korean culture and identity – emphasis on my small eyes, my haraboji's loud trot music emanating through our house, the instances when my mother would speak Korean to me in white spaces. The visceral feeling of these experiences linger, even if my sense of it as an adult has changed.

We imagine that those who grew up like us in a time of the U.S. when Americanized Chinese food (which has a unique history of its own) represented the epitome of "diversity" are likely able to recount similar stories to ours where they grew acutely vigilant of how their race and ethnicity opened them to being othered or even bullied. But, culture evolves, and we can see that what the U.S. culture is today in 2024 and what it co-opts, tolerates, or even grows to superficially accept, shifts the context for Asian Americans. With the popularization of K-pop, pan-Asian cuisines, and Asian culture within white America, Asian Americans are operating in a contemporary sociocultural space where their heritage cultures are viewed as having trending value. Even still, the long-standing stereotypic media portrayals of Asians as foreign threat yet ironically also passive and submissive, exotic, fetishized, cunning, sly, robotic, and unfeeling still linger in this country. The duality of conditional acceptance/underlying hate toward Asian Americans perpetuates anti-Asian sentiment and maintains the power within white supremacy to dictate who and what holds value.

## Transmission of Racism Across Generations

One of the insidious ways in which racism continues to affect families across generations is through members' internalization of it. Acutely aware of social pressures, the second generation often defended against racism by aligning with it through rejecting their family's cultural foods in place of mainstream American food, making the effort to distance themselves from their Asian identity and culture, not making efforts to retain cultural language, and seeking in-membership within white peer circles and non-Asian spaces. These efforts to de-identify with one's Asian heritage and identity were thereby to decrease the potential for social rejection and embarrassment. These processes may not characterize the experiences of all Asian Americans but are heightened for those immersed in white-majority environments with few social connections that are Asian affirming.

Anecdotally, many of us can attest to the fact that the first generation typically did not engage in conversations about racism and discrimination with their children such as parents in other racial groups, like parents in the black community. Research confirms this (Juang et al., 2018). Some may assume that part of the reason is that the immigrant generation assumed that racism was just a part of the reality of immigration. Others might take a cultural view and assume that directly talking about racism and discrimination went against implicit cultural rules in Asian family systems where emotionally vulnerable topics are often not taken as things to discuss between parents and children. Perhaps, another reality might have been that losses around immigration included first-generation parents and second-generation children not sharing a first language to discuss complex matters like this. The first-generation often lacked the English language skills and vocabulary to discuss these matters with their second-generation children who in turn often lacked fluency in the parents' first language. Differences in language significantly affected communication in relationships.

This does not mean that first-generation parents either did not care about trying to protect their children from racism or preparing them to face discrimination. Instead, their efforts to protect and prepare their children were directed more toward tangible actions they thought could offer their children a better future – educational achievement, financial success, and careers with status (Qin et al., 2017). Without directly asking, their emphasis on financial success may have been equally or more about wanting security for their children, rather than the pursuit of wealth or social status. An alternative interpretation of first-generation parenting styles which were perceived to be akin to Chua's (2011) controversial Tiger parenting could be that it was one way that first-generation parents tried to protect. Experiencing the direct reign of white supremacy as immigrants may have shaped beliefs that Asians would always experience discrimination and unequal opportunities within white supremacy's corporate America (Louie, 2004). Thus, emphasizing high grades and motivating their children toward career paths that relied on academic achievement and credentials rather than social capital as the vehicle toward status and success was just as much an effort to help secure a future within a racist society as it was about upholding face (Hsieh, 2021).

## Racism and Mental Health

The continuous witnessing and experiencing of racism and race-based discrimination, fetishization, and violence impacts mental health. This collective trauma can also compound the other forms of trauma that many Asian immigrants may have experienced through war and political violence in their countries of origin. The trauma of war has significant physical consequences like death and loss, injury and disability, loss of livelihoods, equity, and possessions, sexual violence, malnutrition, illness, and emotional ones like anxiety, depression, and PTSD that can be lasting (Murthy & Lakshminarayana, 2006). If war or political violence and its aftermath is the impetus for leaving one's country, that trauma itself can get repressed for a variety of reasons, often to simply survive. Yet, unprocessed trauma continues to impact how one functions mentally, physically, emotionally, and relationally.

Trauma informed perspectives acknowledge how racialized trauma also imprints in our bodies and on our minds, lasting through our DNA (Menakem, 2017). Racialized trauma causes elevated cortisol levels, triggers the fight or flight stress response, and the consequences can be elevated anxiety levels which may present as mood issues, irritability, depression, concentration issues, and social anxiety (Williams & Mohammed, 2009). This is still largely unacknowledged at all systemic levels but may partly explain mental health symptomatology as well as the maladaptive coping strategies one might use, such as substance use (Lei et al., 2021). Yet, without taking this context into consideration, these issues can be mistaken for individual psychopathology.

### Trauma in the Immigrant Experience

When we reflect upon the anecdotal stories and published examples of Asian parents who appear cold, distant, and harsh, we wonder about the context that produces these presentations. However, journal articles and book chapters that speak to parent-child relationships between first-generation Asian immigrants and U.S.-born second-generation children often overlook this context. What results is the assumption that this description simply reflects a cultural way of being, a style of parenting, or individual psycho-emotional issues. We need to use a lens that allows us to capture the humanity in immigration – lives being interrupted, cut-off from countries and relationships that hold attachment, denial of societal membership, and bearing the stresses of everyday life punctuated by marginalization and limited employment options. When this aspect of immigrant parenting is often overlooked or not discussed, Asian American children often narrate their experience of their parents through misunderstanding and resentment.

### Racialized Trauma in Successive Generations

Furthermore, the pressures of trying to survive in a society that was not set up to enable Asian immigrant success can cause one to internalize self-blame and a sense of failure, leading to development of the aforementioned mental health issues. For second and later generation Asian Americans, sometimes the pressure is less about surviving and more about achieving success. The Model Minority Myth (Shih et al., 2019) assumes that the American Dream is attainable. Yet, many do not experience the Dream reality. According to Yip, Gee, and Takeuchi (2008), first-generation immigrants report greater discrimination than the second generation. However, the psycho-emotional impact of discrimination is reported to be more consequential for second-generation persons (Armenta et al., 2013). For U.S.-born Asian Americans, being discriminated against by your own country of birth may be even more disillusioning than when one is rejected by their country of adoption (Huynh et al., 2011). We are American and the connection to this part of our identity is perhaps even more salient than our ethnic heritage, but there are daily reminders that we are seen as un-American.

The pressures that children of immigrant families experience to succeed in order to make their first-generation parents' sacrifices worthwhile can also cause individual mental health problems or relational distress in the parent-child relationship. The pressure of feeling like it is your responsibility to pull your family out of poverty, gain upward mobility, or lift your family's social status through your financial or occupational success can create an overwhelming emotional burden. Even for families who do not experience poverty and financial stress, the ethos of Asian value systems expect the second-generation to succeed and uphold family status and face. Children of immigrants may feel they are a means to an end. These and/or the fear of failure may build resentment, create distancing, and motivate resistance through acts of rebellion (Hsieh, 2021).

As family therapists, we know from Bowenian theory (Kerr & Bowen, 1988) that similar to other family patterns, the consequences of racism can also get passed down through the multigenerational transmission process. Interrupting this process requires awareness and intentional and conscious action.

## We Resist

Many of our families from the first to the second-generation were able to gain upward mobility which can help buffer the impact of racialized stress, discrimination, and racism. However, contrary to the model minority myth, many families also experience ongoing financial stress with marginal improvement over generations (Qin et al., 2017). Therefore, given the diversity of realities that Asian American families experience, it is important to talk about resistance as a range of possibilities. Resistance is multiplicitous, varying from quiet fortitude (ChenFeng et al., 2017) to more active forms of activism. Whether community-based movements and protests, or the day-to-day efforts to move relationships and systems toward equity, regardless of the degree to which our resistance is public facing, it is an underlying aspect of being Asian American.

### Visible Acts of Resistance

Asian Americans have long been considered the "silent minority," but this description handed down by dominant white society is one Asians disprove time and again. Individual examples of stoic endurance exist amid organized, collective actions like the Asian American movement, which united Japanese, Filipino, and Chinese communities whose efforts resulted in adding sufficient pressure to help create ethnic studies programs on college campuses (Wei, 1993), and Asian American activism that added political pressure to help pass the Immigration and Nationality Act (Hong, 2019). The Delano Grape Strike is another powerful example of how Asian Americans effect social change. Filipino American farm workers organized this labor strike in 1965, and it lasted for five years, resulting in a collective bargaining agreement that improved wages and working conditions and eventually helped establish the United Farm Workers (UFW) labor union (Garcia, 2013). After the 1992 L.A. uprisings, Korean and Black tensions increased, playing out a zero-sum game shaped by white supremacist imperialism (Kim, 2021). History remembers how Korean Americans came alongside Black Americans to fight against a white capitalistic system that was pitting communities of color against one another. The sacrifice and efforts of Asian American activists have been too easily swept away under the myth and guise of being "model minority." We are grateful for those who sacrificed and fought to begin the legacy that has continued through Asian American feminist and queer activists who have challenged anti-LGBTQ laws, past and current Asian Americans in solidarity with Black liberation/anti-blackness, and those who continue to stand up for the Stop Asian hate movement. Asian Americans show that the racist trope that we are silent and submissive is inaccurate.

### Activism Based on Relational Process

Other forms of Asian American resistance are practiced daily in less visible but equally powerful ways that highlight the complexity of more subtle forms of resistance across our communities. Resistance in Asian American contexts is nuanced. We protest and raise our voices, and we have also developed our own approaches rooted in relationally rooted values. For example, we know how to apply the relational orientation that we learned from our cultures to build the types of alliances that can move an issue or facilitate change. We also attend to context and adapt our strategies to motivate change because our inherently multicultural socialization enables us to see multiple perspectives, code switch, and code mesh. In addition, claiming the aspects of our identity and existence that society denigrates is also how we take back our power. We unapologetically eat our culture's foods and speak what we know from our family's heritage language, while also engaging in all levels of American life and society as full members of both.

### Countering Internalized Racism

Learning how to counter internalized racism is another critical process of empowerment (Hwang, 2021). My (LK) own journey relates to this. One reality for some second-generation children was being raised in their family's small businesses because their parents typically worked long hours and childcare was either too costly, inaccessible, or infeasible. It certainly was a focal part of my family's story. Much of my time outside of school was spent playing in the aisles of my parents' convenience store, helping replenish shelves, and gleefully eating the inventory.

One of my favorite activities was restocking the soda shelves in the large beverage coolers. As a five-year-old, I would proudly carry two half-gallon bottles tethered together in each hand and follow my dad to each shelf that was running low. I would run around the store and look for other opportunities to lend a hand, and this would not only help to pass the time, but it made me feel useful and capable. My parents took a photo of me holding these soda bottles in my arms, and when it came time for me to submit photos of my childhood to showcase during my high school graduation's family night, I eagerly shared this one. It represented a part of my history, my identity, my family's story of tenacity and survival.

However, I overlooked the fact that this memento may also connect to some aspect of immigrant stigma. I still remember my mother's reaction to seeing this photo displayed on the overhead projector as my name was called for me to cross the stage where all graduates were seated, into the audience to hand roses of appreciation to my loved ones. When I reached her in the audience, she hurriedlywhispered in Korean, "Why would you show that picture?" I did not expect that reaction. In that exchange, I realized that I had highlighted the hard and grueling realities of immigrant life that a first-generation parent might not want shown to others.

Throughout the years, my sense of relational ethics keeps me from asking my mother about her reaction to me that night. I do not want to bring up vulnerability. Nevertheless, I have tried to make sense of that moment. I have two interpretations about this subtext. One is that she just thinks there are better pictures of me in childhood than the one I chose. The other is that she felt internal conflict as a mother about having to raise her children within the walls of her convenience store. While I imagine that she must feel pride about overcoming insurmountable challenges to support her family, she also seems to hold feelings around her low-status work and regret for not having been able to give her children an idealized middle-class childhood she hoped for in the American Dream.

To this day, she often remarks that she could not give us the life that she had wanted to provide. She has never articulated exactly what this means. But, whenever I hear it, I feel a knee-jerk reaction to reassure her that her tireless efforts were more than enough as well as indignation that there is nothing she should have to defend. My parents gave their all and sacrificed everything, like countless other post-1965 Asian immigrants, to provide their children a future of possibilities. I have the deepest sense of awe and respect for my parents at what they were able to accomplish through their sheer determination and hard work as immigrants with little English fluency, no higher education, no social capital, in a racist society. I see how hard they worked and that direct witnessing taught me so much about life and the world. Our story is a living legacy of survival and resilience.

Part of my resistance is owning my family's immigrant history and the realities we lived because of it. I believe that proudly telling these stories, rather than hiding them or being embarrassed about them is a way to resist the internalized racism. So much of the tenacity, grit, creativity, and capability I live out today stems from witnessing my immigrant parents, like many other immigrant parents, toil and overcome countless hardships. By example, they passed down lessons about humility, hard work, determination, integrity, resourcefulness, and hope. Our lives are an extension of their resistance, and we hold privilege to build upon their legacy with our future generations.

## Carrying the Legacy Forward

For second and later generation Asian Americans like us, we do not have to struggle in the exact same ways as the first-generation did because the times and context are different (Kim et al., 2019). Technology connects the world, immigration remains at the forefront of U.S. population growth, and the U.S. takes more multicultural influence. From the Civil Rights Movement of the 1950s and 1960s to racial movements like Black Lives Matter and the 2020–2021 racial unrest following the murder of George Floyd, there is increased racial consciousness in this nation. We owe honor and respect to those who have walked before us and other people of color who created unrest where needed. It is humbling that our children get to grow up in a society that has visible Asian American role models in media (i.e., Steven Yeun, Ali Wong, Jo Koy, Mindy Kaling, etc.) and also see other influencers and affirming reflections of their racial identity (i.e., Vice President Kamala Harris, former CEO of PepsiCo Indra Nooyi, basketball player Jeremy Lin, gymnast Sunisa Lee, celebrity chef Melissa King, etc.). The sociocultural context in 2024 is significantly different than even the era that many of us grew up in during the 1980s and 1990s, and this helps moderate racism.

We also have greater societal power that comes from the privilege of being socialized and educated in the U.S (Kim et al., 2019). The privilege we hold through varying levels of increased educational status, occupational status, economic status, and social status (Hirschman & Wong, 2016) gives us more empowerment to navigate racism. We are the doctors and lawyers that immigrant parents dreamed of, plus we are also leaders, educators, comedians, athletes, creatives, artists, chefs, entrepreneurs, and change agents that are shaping our social context now and into the future. There may still be a lack of Asian American representation in relation to the centrality of whiteness, but we impact all levels of U.S. society, and we take up space. Thus, second and later generations feel more empowered to directly confront racism (Juang et al., 2018).

### Building from Our Privilege to Shape the Future

As parents, the shared language we have with our third-generation children along with our cultural capital enables us to more directly address racism with our children as part of preparing and protecting them (Kim et al., 2019). This means we engage with children about racist experiences and the impact of it when it occurs. We promote open communication to discuss hard topics (Kim et al., 2014). Parents acknowledge their children's experiences, invite them to process it, comfort them, and give them adaptive skills for coping with the hurt, rather than minimizing these experiences. Hwang (2011) proposes that this approach of dealing with racism directly seems to be one of the biggest contrasts from the first-generation who practiced more of an indirect approach around challenging topics.

### Promoting and Engaging Diversity

Many of us recall feeling isolated in our racial identity growing up, so we proactively try to connect our children to diversity. Juang et al. (2018) cite that some make concerted efforts to research the density of Asian Americans in schools and areas where they choose to raise children. Some intentionally seek Asian dense areas due to the assumption that their children may experience less discrimination and thereby decrease some of the protective stress for them as parents. However, if the family lives in predominantly white communities, the parents intentionally socialize their children around discrimination, preparing them to be aware that they are different. They regularly engage in racial socialization and bring up topics relating to diversity and acknowledge that people may judge them because of their race. They help their children resist the internalization of racism by verbally affirming proud aspects of being Asian (Juang et al., 2018).

Second-generation parents see themselves as having greater influence than the first generation did to help impact society (Kim et al., 2019). They also carry forward culturally inspired relational values. Therefore, they make conscious efforts to promote ideas of human equality, diversity beyond race, and embracing differences (Kim et al., 2019). Other forms of proactive racial socialization include reading books about immigration and diversity and educating children about systemic racism, including police brutality rather than waiting for their children to learn about these issues on their own (Juang et al., 2018). They also intentionally seek social connections across identity intersections and integrate their children with families who hold different intersections from themselves. They value diversity, whereas the first-generation tended to reinforce the discrimination they saw as a way to protect their children.

### Claiming Bicultural Identity

Other ways that we carry the legacy forward are through ethnic socialization and our efforts to intentionally pass on heritage traditions that we may also be disconnected from (Kim et al., 2019). This lack of ethnic cultural knowledge might be connected to the racism we encountered and the efforts we made to reject or disassociate from our ethnic heritage. Now, in the U.S. where Asian culture is more accepted by the white mainstream, it can be viewed as "trendy" to eat things like seaweed, moon cakes, or tofu – the foods we were rejected for. Because maintenance of heritage culture already tends to diminish over time, second-generation parents might build community with families from similar ethnic backgrounds, seek out extracurricular language programs, and prioritize time with extended family. We also practice the collectivist values that are deeply ingrained in our identities and ways of relating to others. We nurture both individualistic traits that are social currency in the U.S., while also privileging ethnic values we learned, such as showing respect for elders, attuning to others and how you impact them, and showing generosity and care for the collective.

I (JCF) really resonate with all these tensions of navigating racial identity as my spouse and I parent our two, third-generation Taiwanese American children. Our older child is in his second year of a dual immersion Mandarin program in a public school in a district outside of our home district. Each year we have the conversation around what might continue to be best for his development. One of our primary interests is that in a dual immersion Mandarin program, he will always have at least one teacher who shares his racial/cultural identity, thereby normalizing and centering his foundational identities amongst a racially diverse group of peers. This goes beyond just having an Asian American or Mandarin-speaking teacher, but the cultural values and norms that are taught and celebrated in the classroom and school (Lunar New Year, eating Asian foods, etc.). This is something my spouse and I never had in our years of public education, and we think about the unconscious ways this will allow him to grow up with less minority stress in these formative years because we know the countless racialized realities he will encounter for the rest of his life.

First-generation parents' inclination to focus on family life and their children's upbringing (and less so on the community) is often about surviving in a new country and their racialized experiences of being forgotten and invisibilized. It is hard to engage politically or in community life when there is a disconnect from their own agency and capacity to effect change as racialized peoples. Without examination, we, the second-generation, can default to this posture of life – attending to our own family's concerns in a disconscious way, passing on a self-survival and self-focused existence. It is a privilege to have all this knowledge and awareness about the Asian American experience and with it, we can move in the direction of healing and growth. In doing so, we can live out the next generation of both honoring our elders and their dreams of establishing a good life in the U.S. AND investing in the transformation and liberation of all communities who are oppressed.

## Integrating Migration Legacies in the Therapy Room

Myla was a 38-year-old, second-generation U.S.-born Filipina, middle-SES, cisgender woman, heterosexual, widowed mother who came to therapy for support with anxiety. Myla reported that she had been in therapy once previously, when she was struggling with anxiety during law school. Myla reported that her former therapist focused primarily on helping her build coping skills, but that these skills were inadequately helpful at this time in her life. She looked for a therapist who was also Asian-identified, assuming they might connect based on race. As part of the assessment process, Myla's therapist learned that she worked long hours in a high stakes environment as a corporate lawyer and also carried the stress of managing a busy family life with two young children ages 6 (Owen) and 4 (Oliver) years, plus aging parents who depended on her for general support.

As therapy progressed, the main topic discussed was the intersection of Myla's demanding career and her role as a mother of young children. Recently, Myla described having difficulties with sleep, experiencing low energy, and feeling increasingly overwhelmed by her older son, Owen's, changes in behavior. When the therapist explored this, Myla reported that Owen had become more emotionally sensitive, harder to soothe when upset, and that his bedtime routine had become a struggle. She acknowledged that because she already experienced difficulties balancing all of her roles, the new struggles significantly raised the anxiety she felt around her mothering responsibilities. Myla also talked about new roles she was taking on at work and how she felt like the compounding stress of work and home life were leading to burnout.

The therapist asked Myla about her sense of what might be affecting Owen's behavioral and emotional changes. They explored potential individual factors, and after ruling out medical and developmental changes, they turned to environmental and social contexts. When the therapist asked about school, Myla said that Owen was four months into his first-grade year at the same school where he had completed Kindergarten. She perceived him as feeling connected to his teacher, making friends, and adjusting well. When reflecting on the home environment, Myla noted that due to her increased work responsibilities, her work that she could not just leave at the office was spilling over even more into life after-hours. When home with her kids, she often had to respond to emails, take calls, and split her attention. She continued to rely on childcare support from her mother when her mother felt physically well, her father, and mother-in-law who remained active in their lives even after Myla's husband's death three years ago.

The therapist asked about the school that Owen attended and asked about the school culture and about the racial/ethnic/class diversity. As a small, non-religious private school, there was a smaller teacher-to-student ratio and many of the families were well connected. There was a sense of community, and this was one of the reasons why Myla had chosen this school. However, Myla lived in a white majority neighborhood, and Owen's school had limited racial/ethnic/class diversity, too.

Not wanting to overemphasize the salience of any one part of Myla's identity, or assume either Myla's sense of ethnic identity or pathologize a potential lack of this, the therapist broadly wondered about Myla's experience of self in community context. The therapist explored if it was notable for Myla and her family to live in a mostly white neighborhood and community by asking what types of neighborhoods the family was used to living in and how their neighborhood felt to live in. Myla reported that they had mostly lived in white neighborhoods and that this mirrored her childhood, too. She reported friendly and close relationships with a few of the families in her neighborhood who had children the same age. The therapist also explored the role of cultural heritage and whether or not this was a salient aspect of Myla's identity and her children's identities. She responded that her connection to her Filipino heritage was mostly experienced through her parents and some close family friends who she regarded as her "aunties" and "uncles." She expressed a close connection to culture through food and the large, holiday gatherings her parents and their friends hosted during Easter and Thanksgiving.

When the therapist asked about Myla's experience of her professional identity and status within her family context, she learned that Myla's professional status represented upward cultural and economic mobility to her family. Myla's parents were both college educated and they had both been registered nurses in their hometown of Cebu City in the Philippines, but only her mother was able to secure a job in residential nursing after they immigrated to Oregon in the early 1980s. Myla's father did the bulk of caregiving for Myla and her older brother until he took a job in a meat processing plant where he worked until his retirement. Myla recalled regular conflict in her parents' relationship that related to the family's financial instability and stress in the first ten years after they immigrated. As a part of this conversation, Myla referred to herself as a "rule follower" and explained that part of that was out of intentions to keep her parents from worrying about her because she was already acutely aware of how much stress they always seemed to carry.

Myla noted that her law school acceptance had been a "big deal" to her parents and that she knew this because of how much she heard it come up in conversations whenever her parents were at social gatherings with their Filipino friends. While she felt a general sense of interest and reward in the work she did as a corporate lawyer, she also commented on the level of pressure she experienced in it. Myla explained that her field was highly competitive and that getting her foot in the door had taken lots of strategic networking and climbing of the professional ladder in a historically white male-dominated specialty. At the content level, Myla was responsible for helping her company manage systems connected to multimillion dollar budgets, and at the relational level, Myla had to manage complex everyday office politics of a corporate workplace as a petite, Filipina American woman. Myla always felt like her professional status could be threatened and the high performance level she had to maintain in order to keep her job. She was also very conscious of her role as the sole financial provider for her family and that she had to be the safety net for her parents as they aged. There was little margin for error.

The therapist was curious whether Myla's anxiety reflected any relationship between the pressure to carry multiple high stakes roles and the potential of underlying migration stress Myla might be carrying around her own unnamed marginalized identities in her neighborhood and workplace as well as her parents' marginalization as immigrants. The therapist asked Myla how she managed the level of performance pressure that she carried. Myla responded that she just held it in and the therapist asked metaphorically if it felt sort of like she was holding her breath while frantically trying to keep her head above water. Myla nodded her head in agreement and said that it felt like if she made a mistake, everything would fall apart for the people who depended on her. She asked the therapist if this just meant she was a perfectionist like some of her friends had said.

The therapist challenged this superficial and misattributed idea by acknowledging that perfectionism could be one perspective but punctuated Myla's second-generation context, saying that she believed Myla was more likely functioning the way she was because there was a system that warranted it. She went on to ask, what currents could be pushing against her that made her have to swim so frantically while holding her breath. The therapist explained that she heard Myla referring to very real sociocultural factors that powerfully affected the context within which she lived and functioned as a petite, Filipina, cisgender woman, corporate lawyer in a white male-dominant workplace, single mother to young children, and adult child of immigrant Filipino aging parents.

The therapist validated Myla's anxiety given the level of relational and occupational pressure she experienced, and then used a socioculturally attuned lens (Knudson-Martin, Kim, Gibbs, & Harmon, 2021) to deconstruct her felt vulnerability in the context of invisible minority stress and survival stress that might relate to her immigrant parents' multigenerational migration legacy. Through this lens, the therapist helped Myla depathologize the anxiety as individual perfectionistic tendencies and instead see it as part of how she was unknowingly carrying her family's migration legacy forward. The therapist affirmed Myla's resilience and the resilience her family had demonstrated through their immigrant struggle, but facilitated attention to the ways Myla and her parents' context were also different. Highlighting Myla's second-generation identity, native English ability, and increased occupational, social, cultural, and economic capital, the therapist helped Myla explore how she was able to move through the world differently than her first-generation parents and counter discrimination and racism in society and in the workplace differently than her parents had been able to. She did this while also acknowledging the very real climate of racism that continued to explicitly and implicitly impact her and her family.

This conversation led to discussing internalized racism which the therapist normalized as an inadvertent and common result of the racism and minority stress Asian Americans experience. They discovered that one of the survival mechanisms that Myla had developed was to minimize the racist experiences she witnessed her parents have that she also had. Because her parents coped with racism by accepting it and acting like it did not matter, they also did not address it when Myla reported the racist things kids would say to her. Myla said, "Instead of discussing it with me, my parents showed they cared by making my favorite foods when I had painful experiences that I would share as a child. I sort of do the same with my kids, too." Tangible acts of care like this reflect common cultural strategies used around emotion in Asian American families.

Myla learned to connect how her tendency to minimize and overlook issues in her life and her children's lives that did not rise to a crisis level connected to her internalized family migration legacy of survival. Myla then connected that this might be contributing to the changes she was seeing in her older son, Owen. She explained that Owen had come home from school a couple of months ago asking why his nose looked "different" and expressing hurt that kids had made fun of him and told him his nose was "flat." She stated that she told him to ignore what the kids had said. She saw that dismissing his hurt and ignoring this racism mirrored how her parents tended to handle it with her as a child, saying things like, "That's (racist comment about shape of nose) not something to cry about. Just be grateful you have a nose to breathe and smell through." She knew these statements were to help, but she saw how complacent they were, which reflected their silent fortitude and lack of social and cultural capital as first-generation immigrants. She now recognized these moments were opportunities to act from a different context to expand her family's repertoire for claiming their membership in American society. Therapeutic conversations continued to shift from narratives around survival to transformative narratives of sustainability beyond survival.

## Writing the Next Chapter in Migration Legacies

As therapists, we know that telling one's story and what gets punctuated versus what gets omitted, all matter in having the ability to author and re-author the future (White & Epston, 1990). The way we discuss the trauma held in family migration legacies in this chapter does not account for the ways that important individual and family factors, circumstances, and events mediate immigration legacies. These require additional attention and should be considered. Systemically, it affects a family's context, its way of functioning, and relational dynamics. However, here we propose that discussing migration legacies is also needed to write the next chapter of a family's life.

We know the migration story starts long before the actual leaving takes place. The decision to immigrate and the process it takes is complex. In Asian family contexts, this decision is most likely a collective one with considerations about who leaves, who stays, and how to stay connected across the distance. There is uncertainty to navigate and the process to immigrate can be long and entail financial, emotional, and relational sacrifices from the family. But, the resulting realities on both sides are not fully felt or known until long after the departure. The post-immigration experience can also include managing the lingering impacts of trauma, complicated grief, and ambiguous loss (Boss, 2009) held within the psyche of many Asian American families.

Immigration is not a single event. It is a story that continues through each generation. Yet, this story can either be told in a one-dimensional way, simply not discussed, or intentionally kept in a shroud of silence. What keeps families from discussing their migration histories in more personal and multifaceted ways? A discussion regarding the various reasons for the explicit silence is a complex topic of its own and one that is beyond the scope of this chapter. But, a common version of the immigration story many of us know is the single story that the first generation came for a better life and future for the next generation. Yet, that is only part of the story. A second-generation Asian American research participant once admitted to me that she felt some irritation whenever her parents would cite that reason because she did not believe her parents were merely self-sacrificing. She rhetorically said,

> C'mon. They're human. I mean, would you give up everything you know, take on these huge risks and unknowns, to live the hard life they had to here? Who would do that? They had to have assumed they would also benefit in some way. I've always believed there's more to the story.

So, beyond the version we hear, what else can be said and what makes it important to say?

We believe it is important to tell stories held within and about our family migration legacies because these hold values, lessons, and meanings that provide context for identity and relationship building. The stories shared may highlight aspects that reflect obvious strength and pride, but the more vulnerable parts may be even more healing to share and foster resilience and deeper connection. Relational repair is facilitated when we can know the first generation beyond the linear descriptions that can get produced. Furthermore, when we know our history, we are able to thread together more complete versions of ourselves to carry forward into how we live.

## Reflection Questions

### Questions for the Therapist

- What is the migration narrative told in your family? How did you learn about it? Who tells it and what gets told? What aspects are held back? What might be meaningful to learn more about?
- Where do you locate yourself in your family's migration narrative? How do you tell it?
- How do the models for navigating racism that you saw in your family get played out in your life today? How do you maintain it? Should you shift it? How do you shift it?
- How does being second or later generation influence the context of possibilities for your sustainability today?

### Questions for Therapy

- I wonder how differences in migration status between you and your parents might affect the range of options available to you that would not have been available to your parents in this situation?

- What aspects of internalized racism might be affecting the approach you are taking in this situation? How might it be holding you back? How might it be keeping you from seeing other possibilities?
- What are the values and qualities you witnessed and learned from your family migration legacy that you continue to demonstrate today? What makes maintaining this narrative meaningful to you? Meaningful to others?

## References

Armenta, B. E., Lee, R. M., Pituc, S. T., Jung, K-R., Park, I. M. K., Soto, J. A., & Schwartz, S. J. (2013). Where are you from? A validation of the Foreigner Objectification Scale and the psychological correlates of foreigner objectification among Asian Americans and Latinos. *Cultural Diversity and Ethnic Minority Psychology, 19*, 131–142. https://doi.org/10.1037/a0031547

Boss, P. (2009). The trauma and complicated grief of ambiguous loss. *Pastoral Psychology, 59*, 137–145. https://doi.org/10.1007/s11089-009-0264-0

Budiman, A., & Ruiz, N. G. (2021). Asian Americans are the fastest-growing racial or ethnic group in the US. https://www.pewresearch.org/short-reads/2021/04/09/asian-americans-are-the-fastest-growing-racial-or-ethnic-group-in-the-u-s/

ChenFeng, J., Kim, L., Knudson-Martin, C., & Wu, Y. (2017). Addressing culture, gender, and power with Asian American couples: Application of socio-emotional relationship therapy. *Family Process, 56*(3), 558–573. https://doi.org/10.1111/famp.12251

Chua, A. (2011). *Battle hymn of the tiger mother.* Penguin Books.

Garcia, M. (2013). A moveable feast: The UFW grape boycott and farm worker justice. *International Labor and Working-Class History, 83*(83), 146–153. https://doi.org/10.1017/S0147547913000021

Gover, A. R., Harper, S. B., & Langton, L. (2020). Anti-Asian Hate crime during the COVID-19 pandemic: Exploring the reproduction of inequality. *American Journal of Criminal Justice, 45*(4), 647–667. https://doi.org/10.1007/s12103-020-09545-1

Hirschman, C., & Wong, M. G. (2016). Trends in socioeconomic achievement among immigrant and native-born Asian-Americans, 1960–1976. *The Sociological Quarterly, 22*(4), 495–514. https://doi.org/10.1111/j.1533-8525.1981.tb00677.x

Hong, J.H. (2019). *Opening the gates to Asia: A transpacific history of how America repealed Asian exclusion.* University of North Carolina Press.

Hsieh, N. (2021). *Constructing bicultural identity and shame resilience in Chinese Americans* [Doctoral dissertation, Loma Linda University].

Huynh, Q. L., Devos, T., & Smalarz, L. (2011). Perpetual foreigner in one's own land: Potential implications for identity and psychological adjustment. *Journal of Social and Clinical Psychology, 30*(2), 133–162. https://doi.org/10.1521/jscp.2011.30.2.133.

Hwang, W.-C. (2011). Acculturative family distancing. In F. Leong, L. Juang, D. B. Qin, & H. E. Fitzerald (Eds.), *Asian American and Pacific Islander children and mental health* (Vol. 1, pp. 47–70). ABC-CLIO.

Hwang, W.-C. (2021). Demystifying and addressing internalized racism and oppression among Asian Americans. *American Psychologist, 76*(4), 596–610. https://doi.org/10.1037/amp0000798

Juang, L. P., Park, I., Kim, S. Y., Lee, R. M., Qin, D., Okazaki, S., Swartz, T. T., & Lau, A. (2018). Reactive and proactive ethnic-racial socialization practices of second-generation Asian American parents. *Asian American Journal of Psychology, 9*(1), 4–16. https://doi.org/10.1037/aap0000101

Kerr, M. E., & Bowen, M. (1988). *Family evaluation* (1st ed.). W.W. Norton & Company.

Kim, L., Knudson-Martin, C., & Tuttle, A. (2019). Transmission of intergenerational migration legacies in Korean American families: Parenting the third generation. *Contemporary Family Therapy*, 41, 180-190. https://doi.org/10.1007/s10591-018-9485-7

Kim, L., Knudson-Martin, C., & Tuttle, A. (2014). Torward relationship-directed parenting: An example of North American born second-generation Korean-American mothers and their partners. *Family Process*, 53, 55-66. 10.1111/famp.12052

Kim, N. (2021, April 21). The unexpected alliance forged after the Rodney King verdict. *The Washington Post.*

Knudson-Martin, C., Kim, L., Gibbs, E., & Harmon, R. (2021). Sociocultural attunement to vulnerability in couple therapy: Fulcrum for changing power processes in heterosexual relationships. *Family Process, 60*(4), 1152–1169. https://doi.org/10.1111/famp.12635

Lee, E. (2015). *The Making of Asian American.* Simon & Schuster.

Lei, Y., Shah, V., Biely, C., Jackson, N., Dudovitz, R., Barnert, E., Hotez, E., Guerrero, A., Bui, A. L., Sastry, N., & Schickedanz, A. (2021). Discrimination and subsequent mental health, substance use, and well-being in young adults. *Pediatrics, 148*(6), 1–10. https://doi.org/10.1542/peds.2021-051378

Li, Y., & Nicholson, H.L. Jr. (2021). When "model minorities" become "yellow peril": Othering and the racialization of Asian Americans in the COVID-19 pandemic. *Social Compass, 15*(2):e12849. https://doi.org/10.1111/soc4.12849

Louie, V. S. (2004). *Compelled to excel: Immigration, education, and opportunity among Chinese Americans.* Stanford University Press.

McClain, C. J. (1994). *In search of equality: The Chinese struggle against discrimination in 19th-century America.* University of California Press.

Menakem, R. (2017). *My grandmother's hands: Racialized trauma and the pathway to mending our hearts and bodies.* Central Recovery Press.

Murthy, R. S., & Lakshminarayanam R. (2006). Mental health consequences of war: A brief review of research findings. *World Psychiatry, 5*(1), 25–30.

Qin, D. B., Chang, T., Xie, M., Liu, S., & Rana, M. (2017). Socioeconomic status and child/youth outcomes in Asian American families. In Y. Choi, & H. Hahm (Eds.), *Asian American parenting: culture, family process, and youth development* (pp. 89–115). Springer Publishing Company.

Shih, K. Y., Chang, T. F., & Chen, S. Y. (2019). Impacts of the model minority myth on Asian American individuals and families: Social justice and critical race feminist perspectives. *Journal of Family Theory & Review, 11*(3), 412–428. https://doi.org/10.1111/jftr.12342

Tuan, M. (1998). *Forever foreigners or honorary whites? The Asian ethnic experience today.* Rutgers University Press.

Wei, W. (1993). *The Asian American movement.* Temple University Press

White, M., & Epston, D. (1990). *Narrative means to therapeutic ends* (1st ed.). W.W. Norton & Company.

Williams, D. R., & Mohammed, S. A. (2009). Discrimination and racial disparities in health: Evidence and needed research. *Journal of Behavioral Medicine, 32*(1), 20–47. https://doi.org/10.1007/S10865-008-9185-0

Yip, T., Gee, G. C., & Takeuchi, D. T. (2008). Racial discrimination and psychological distress: The impact of ethnic identity and age among immigrant and United States-born Asian adults. *Developmental Psychology, 44*(3), 787–800. https://doi.org/10.1037/0012-1649.44.3.787

Zhou, M., & Kim, S. S. (2006). Community forces, social capital, and educational achievement: The case of supplementary education in the Chinese and Korean immigrant communities. *Harvard Educational Review, 76,* 1–23. https://doi.org/10.17763/haer.76.1.u08t548554882477

# Chapter 6

# Therapy as Activism

## Transforming Therapy Spaces and Healing Communities

*Ulash Thakore-Dunlap and Bowbay Liang-Hua Feng*

This chapter will focus on the role of marriage and family therapists (MFTs) as activists in creating healing therapeutic spaces for Asian Americans in therapy. As Asian American identified therapists, we define healing therapeutic spaces as those where therapists help to reduce barriers for clinical care, support their clients, explore ways to dismantle systemic oppressive structures within their clinical work and settings, and continually engage in learning more about Asian American mental health. Specifically, this chapter will explore how as authors, we define transformative therapy as activism, what it means for MFTs to engage in activism in therapy, and frameworks used to support Asian American clients. A case example has been provided to illustrate how activism shows up in therapy and clinical techniques helpful for this work.

## Meaning of Transformative Therapy as Activism

Transformative therapy as activism is an active choice therapists make in commitment to addressing social injustices and systemic inequalities within the therapeutic process. We recognize that mental health and well-being are not isolated from societal issues and that therapy can be a platform for empowerment and social change. As authors, we believe it is important to share what it personally means to engage in transformative therapy as activism and connect to the topic before delving into the frameworks we use to support our Asian American clients.

### Bowbay

I am a licensed marriage and family therapist (LMFT) and a multiracial Asian American. My unique background is a mix of Chinese, Norwegian, German, Irish, English, and Native American, and growing up in California and living and working internationally. These diverse experiences have shaped who I am today and my belief that individual identities are multifaceted and need to be understood within the broader systemic context. During my formative years, I

DOI: 10.4324/9781003321590-9

often faced bullying and had to navigate the complexities of multiple cultural spaces. This journey led me to understand the importance of holding multiple perspectives at once. I learned to hold a strong sense of belonging and culture as well as acknowledging the truth of exclusion and racism. These personal experiences have been instrumental in shaping my therapeutic approach. I have also had the privilege as part-time faculty to teach graduate courses in counseling psychology. I helped students navigate their own identities and understand the significance of a multicultural lens in the field of counseling psychology. Now, in my private practice, I am passionate about helping people explore their intersectional identities. I place a strong focus on mindfulness, meditation, trauma healing, and compassion. I see therapy as a healing space where clients can embark on a journey to become their authentically integrated selves.

To me, engaging in transformative therapy as activism is deeply personal. It is about recognizing that every therapy session is an opportunity not just to heal individuals but to challenge the very systems that have caused harm. As someone deeply committed to this approach, I see it as a chance to make a difference, not just in my clients' lives but in the world at large. It means being an advocate, a listener, and a change agent all at once. It is about acknowledging that mental health does not exist in a vacuum, but is deeply intertwined with the fabric of society. For me, this means understanding the struggles that marginalized individuals face and helping them heal from the wounds of systemic oppression and discrimination. It is a reminder that, as therapists, we have a role to play in dismantling oppressive systems and making the world a more just place.

### Ulash

I am a licensed marriage and family therapist (LMFT) in California and identify as South Asian, specifically Asian Indian heritage. I was born in London, UK, to a working-class Asian Indian immigrant family. I grew up in a predominantly white working-class community, and from an early age I experienced racism. In my community and the schools I attended in the UK, I felt so helpless that I did not have a voice and could not help others who experienced racism. From an early age, I knew I wanted to get out of poverty as a first-generation Asian Indian and wanted to be in a field where I could support and advocate for others.

While working as an educator and counselor for over 20 years, I have observed the lack of access to education and mental health services for students of color and their families, and the need for advocacy and activism. I see advocacy as something I do every day in my personal and professional life in supporting others to have a voice and access to education and mental resources. In my clinical work with Asian American clients, I provide a space to allow my clients to unpack their narratives of what it means to be Asian and Asian American and ways racism impacts their mind, body, and spirit. Professionally, I am engaged in advocacy at a local and national level on increasing education and mental health access and resources for communities of color. Specifically, my clinical work centers on supporting Asian Americans and ensuring all Asian American groups are represented in the Asian narrative. Currently, as an advocacy effort and passion of mine, I am the senior editor of the first book published on counseling and psychology for South Asian Americans, a group that tends to be marginalized from the Asian American narrative (Nadal, 2019).

## MFTs Engaging in Activism in Supporting Their Asian American Clients

MFTs engaging in activism includes the work that is conducted within and outside of clinical sessions. In the clinical context, focus can be on both micro and macro steps. Micro steps (Holyoak et al., 2021) refer to processes that can help clients have a voice and feel validated. For example, these can include helping clients explore ways to have a voice within their families and manage the stress in their work settings (Holyoak et al., 2021). Macro steps can include discussions about the social actions one can engage in, such as protesting, supporting organizations financially, addressing systemic racism at work (Williams et al., 2022a), and writing to their local and national legislators about an issue the client is concerned about (Holyoak et al., 2021). It is important for therapists to share with clients that there is no right or wrong way to be an advocate or activist, and not all clients are ready to take macro steps in advocating outside of their clinical sessions.

The American Association for Marriage and Family Therapy (AAMFT) code of ethics calls its members to provide services to individuals without discriminating based on race and ethnicity (AAMFT, 2015). The California Association for Marriage and Family Therapists (CAMFT) code of ethics has an additional part to include being aware of and to not perpetuate historical and/or social prejudices when working with clients (CAMFT, 2019). Therefore, part of one's MFT activism involves engaging in trainings on antiracism, understanding the barriers to treatment for Asian Americans, and understanding the nuances and diversity of Asian Americans within the United States such as anti-Asian hate and impact on client's mental health during COVID-19 (Cheng et al., 2021; Nadal, 2018; Williams et al., 2022b).

Furthermore, greater consciousness is needed about the general lack of representation of certain Asian American groups. Since the Asian American Movement, Filipino Americans, South Asian Americans, and Southeast Asian Americans have vocalized feelings of marginalization and exclusion within the pan-ethnic group (Nadal, 2019). For example, the field of South Asian American counseling is still a growing field that needs further advocacy, attention, resources, and visibility devoted to Brown Asian Americans. More training is needed for working with South Asian American clients (Thakore-Dunlap et al., 2023).

Both of us are aware of the experience of holding multiple experiences, and many Asian Americans hold multiple identities. Multiracial people comprise the fastest-growing racial group in the nation and are expected to make up over 10% of the United States population by 2060 (U.S. Census Bureau, 2018). For therapists working with multiracial Asian American clients, Root's (1990) model of multiracial identity development can be helpful. This model proposes four multiracial identity possibilities: acceptance of the identity society assigns, identification of both racial groups, identification of a single racial group, or identification of a new racial group.

Identity can also be fluid and influenced by the environment or context. The pressures from family, geographic location, and the intensity of oppression all shape racial identity development. Although multiracial Asian/white youth perceive less racial discrimination than monoracial Asians, they still experience greater discrimination than monoracial white youth. Several studies link these experiences of discrimination to negative mental health outcomes for multiracial persons (Salahuddin & O'Brien, 2011; Yoo et al., 2016). In addition to racial stress, other challenges may include familial discrimination, and racial identity invalidation, such as individuals imposing an inaccurate racial categorization onto them (Franco et al., 2021).

## Frameworks in Supporting Transformative Therapeutic Spaces for Asian Americans

Texts, theories, and clinical practices in the field of MFT and counseling continue to center around European and white norms (Erolin & Wieling, 2020; Moss & Singh, 2015; Singh et al., 2020). To promote a clinical understanding of communities of color, pedagogical strategies need to encourage critical thinking and promote awareness of the systemic oppression of communities of color (Sharma & Hipolito-Delgado, 2021). There are numerous decolonizing frameworks which center on communities of color experiences to better help, support, and understand Asian American clinical needs. Critical Race Theory (CRT), specifically AsianCrit, are frameworks that can help therapists understand how racialized experiences impact the well-being of Asian American clients, facilitate meaning-making around one's histories and narratives, and elevate client voices in the therapeutic process. We use these frameworks both to understand ways that race and racism impact Asian Americans and to support transformative therapeutic spaces.

### Critical Race Theory (CRT) and AsianCrit

Asian Americans deal with discrimination, racism, and race-based stress, which negatively impact their mental health (Hall & Yee, 2012). In the context of transformative therapy as activism, therapists aim to support clients in challenging and healing from the impact of systemic oppression, discrimination, and trauma. CRT recognizes that racism is embedded in our power structures and woven into our everyday lives through the education system, laws, work settings, and health care and mental health settings, all of which advantage white individuals given that cultural norms are centered around whiteness (Delgado & Stefancic, 2017; Ladson-Billings & Tate, 1995; Moodley et al., 2018). CRT encourages elevating counter-narratives of communities of color as a strategy to counter dominant white discourses and elevate underrepresented voices (Moodley et al., 2018).

AsianCrit builds upon CRT and focuses on ways that race and racism impact the lives and identities of Asian Americans living in the United States (Iftikar & Museus, 2018; Museus & Iftikar, 2013), and this can be used in conjunction with CRT. AsianCrit has helped us (Bowbay and Ulash) to understand the challenges Asian Americans encounter, such as the experience of being seen as foreigners in the United States, the impact of colonialism on identities and experiences, the impact of racial oppression, that Asians are not a monolithic group, and the ways intersectionality (e.g., race, gender, social class) creates unique experiences for Asian Americans (Museus & Iftikar, 2013). Such experiences can negatively impact mental health leading to depression, anxiety, and suicide (Duldulao et al., 2009). Asian Americans may also experience somatization disorder characterized by symptoms of fearfulness, irritability, and a heavy feeling in the chest (Sue & Sue, 1999). In the therapy room, taking an AsianCrit approach validates what is often not named and gives voice to the Asian American experience that is deeply and often painfully known. Having this context reduces shame and gives a landscape to understand racial oppression in the United States for Asian Americans. Therefore, using AsianCrit can help therapists to take a decolonizing approach to therapy to address ways systems of colonization, oppression, and racism have had an impact on clients and on their mental health and well-being.

## The Role of Spirituality and Traditional Healing

The protective and healing role of spirituality is a key resource for both of us (Ulash and Bowbay) in our work with clients and in our personal lives. We use our understanding of our traditional practices, such as honoring our ancestors, to make connections to how healing such practices can be in using the wisdom and strength of our ancestors to create change to support us as therapists so we can better support our clients.

We encourage therapists to create space to explore and understand the many complex intersectional beliefs that Asian American clients may have regarding spirituality and traditional healing practices. Indigenous healing and spiritual practices are used by some Asian Americans and include traditional healers through religious leaders and community leaders (APA, 2012). Some Asian Americans may identify as religious but not practicing and define themselves as spiritual and identify with the principles and beliefs of religion without connecting to an organized religion (Fogelin, 2007). For South

Asian Americans, such religious and spiritual practices have direct connections to the cultural practices and norms that are passed through generations in the South Asian American community (Panchal & Alif, 2023). For some of our clients it may be a deep connection to nature.

Religion and spirituality can be protective factors for the development of psychological distress among Asian Americans (APA, 2012). Therefore, understanding the role of religion, spirituality, and traditional healers for clients can be helpful information in incorporating into the clinical treatment in supporting Asian American clients. It can also be a strong base for community support and connection.

## Clinical Case Example: Jasmine

Asian American identities are diverse, and context such as where a person geographically resides, their racial identity, socioeconomic status, and family migration patterns impacts how individuals maneuver and engage with others. The case of Jasmine provides a clinical case example and overview of how therapists might approach supporting clients navigating their racial identity and racism, specifically anti-Asian hate experiences.

Jasmine identifies as a 48-year-old Vietnamese American, cisgender female. Jasmine sought out working with an Asian American female therapist in March 2021 in a private practice setting. Jasmine shared during the first session having a negative experience with her past therapist "She (the past therapist) did not understand my experiences of being a second-generation Vietnamese American woman, and how important my family and spirituality are to me." Jasmine's parents fled Vietnam as refugees and established life on the east coast working as doctors at a large hospital. Jasmine moved from the east coast to California for her undergraduate studies in engineering and has since stayed, currently residing in San Jose, California. In the first therapy session, Jasmine reports being close to her parents and siblings, is deeply connected to her Vietnamese and American history and culture, is very spiritual, and attends her temple regularly which is a huge source of support.

Jasmine came to therapy after experiencing some anti-Asian hate crimes during the pandemic. Jasmine works for a large tech firm in the San Francisco Bay Area. During March 2020, Jasmine was working remotely and had to go back to the office in January 2021, which is when she started to experience being taunted in public with verbal assault. She was yelled at and called "China flu" and told, "This is your fault, go home." Due to these experiences, Jasmine was afraid to take public transportation to work for fear of being targeted and attacked because of her race. In the first therapy session, Jasmine also expressed being worried for her Asian identified neighbors, friends, and temple members. At work, Jasmine shared feeling unsupported and misunderstood by her colleagues and boss around the anti-Asian hate experiences. Jasmine feels her colleagues dismiss her comments, leaving her feeling minimized. Because of these race-based verbal attacks and the lack of support, Jasmine has been experiencing anxiety, trouble sleeping, anger and frustration, and isolation, all of which impact her well-being. Jasmine also shares feeling powerlessness in not being able to do anything to stop the anti-Asian hate from occurring.

### Treatment Process

Given that Jasmine shared her negative past therapeutic experiences where her racialized experiences were minimized, the therapist who identifies as South Asian American felt it was essential in the first clinical session to build rapport with Jasmine by honoring her past experiences in therapy of not feeling heard and supporting Jasmine around her racial identity. The therapist also explores Jasmine's hopes for working with an Asian American therapist.

#### Coping with Race-Based Stressors

In the clinical sessions, the therapist learns Jasmine is experiencing race-based stress as she has been the target of racist slurs while using public transportation to get to work, microaggressions in the workplace, all of which have caused anxiety, fear, and stress. The therapist provided clinical space to listen to Jasmine's experiences around these events and to share her feelings of fear, shame, and feeling alone. The therapist remained curious by asking open questions, such as "Tell me more about feeling shame and fear." Anti-Asian stereotyping and racism are prevalent in the United States, and many Asian Americans have come from countries that have a history of colonization. Therefore, acknowledging racism and validating the negative impact of the current political and social climate by naming the internalization and external oppression is an important clinical microstep (Chopra, 2021). The therapist also uses psychoeducation to help Jasmine contextualize her experiences as an Asian American given the legacy of Asian racism in the United States, and help her to not feel alone in her experience (Lee & Waters, 2021).

The therapist also validates Jasmine's experiences of anxiety and fear as a result of the racism and explores ways Jasmine has been coping. In the clinical sessions, the therapist uses a trauma-informed lens to explain what racism does to the nervous system. Understanding the nervous system helps clients have agency (Dana, 2020). In therapy sessions, the therapist uses mindfulness techniques to help Jasmine regulate her emotions and nervous system. Inviting Jasmine to notice her feelings while staying connected to her feet and naming the objects in the room helps her to be with hard feelings and be grounded in the present safe environment. The therapist also uses meditation techniques such as visualizations, focusing on the breath and body to help Jasmine feel more grounded and less anxious. Teaching grounding and stabilizing techniques helps clients to increase safety, connection, and choice (Dana, 2020; Menakem, 2017;

Van der Kolk, 2014). In sessions, Jasmine shares how helpful mindfulness techniques have been in "quieting my mind and feeling less anxious."

I (Bowbay) often share with my clients what I learned from my mentor and what has helped me in my own journey. I encourage my clients to hold on to their own stories, to take the time to listen to their own hearts, and the resilience that has been passed down to them – that resonates for them. I say, "hold onto your own story, throughout life others will try to tell you what your story is, do not let them, hold on to who you are." Many of us have had experiences of others telling us who we are and are not, who we can be or not, or what we should be and have been faced by those with entitlement who believe you should fit in the box that is easiest for them, regardless of your experience. Many of my clients have shared stories of being told "you are not enough or aren't you really just…," or the classic dysconscious question often asked, "what are you?" Therapy as activism creates a space of safety, acceptance, and validation, a place to write and own our story. Being able to compassionately explore with respectful curiosity what we are feeling and believing is powerful.

Watts-Jones (2002) noted that, "transforming the pain and shame of internalized racism requires us to look deeply and be present with it, in silence and in voice. Witnessing our pain with the eyes of compassion is healing" (p. 594). For many it is a new experience to reclaim their story and to acknowledge all the stories we have collected that are undigested and not ours. Mindfulness is done through being present in the moment versus being engaged in thoughts in the past or future, curious to understand versus reacting, accepting of what is versus what we wish the situation was. In this way, non-judgmental exploration creates awareness of old patterns that may be a part of generational trauma and supports a client to navigate and understand their own narrative. We have often seen clients shift to a place of stronger agency and understanding.

### Supporting Jasmine's Cultural and Racial Identity

In clinical sessions, Jasmine shares that having a strong Asian identity is deeply connected to her Vietnamese and American history and culture, and she attends her temple regularly. Jasmine expresses her anger and frustration around the increase in anti-Asian hate crimes and impact it has had on her and the community. Jasmine states feeling powerless in not being able to do anything to stop the hate crimes from occurring. Jasmine discusses the microaggressions she experiences both in and out of the workplace that seem to coincide with the increase in anti-Asian hate at large. Given that Jasmine strongly identifies as being Vietnamese American, the therapist felt it important to explore Jasmine's culture and racial identity and how the anti-Asian hate experiences might be impacting her. In providing space to explore Jasmine's cultural and racial identity in therapy, it provided a space for Jasmine to be proud of her Asian identity during a time when Jasmine feels attacked for her race and culture, particularly by her white colleagues. Jasmine shares she is feeling anger and frustration toward all white individuals, particularly her white manager who continues to dismiss Jasmine's comments when she mentions her experiences of racism. This seems to mirror the process described during the immersion stage of Helms's (1990) People of Color Racial Identity model whereby fear, anger, and distrust of white people can grow in the face of repeated experiences such as the ones Jasmine has had of racism. As an act of her resilience, Jasmine is proud that recent racist incidents have not changed her strong Asian American identity. Over several sessions, the therapist works with Jasmine by providing space to process and feel her emotions around these attacks.

Commonly, clients of color in the immersion stage seek out someone of a similar racial and cultural background, such as what Jasmine did, to feel validated in racialized experiences (Tatum, 2003). Jasmine shared in clinical sessions how helpful it was to work with an Asian-identified therapist. The therapist supports and nurtures Jasmine's Asian American identity at this time by helping her identify activities that will help affirm this part of her identity. Jasmine recognizes that it will help her to stay active with her temple attendance, engagement with community activities, and reach out more to her Asian American friends who she has not seen much since the pandemic. To support Jasmine's experience with microaggressions, the therapist helps her plan out how she might address them in the workplace, such as finding allies for support and validation, reporting occurrences if needed to human resources, and keeping documentation of the discrimination she experiences. Jasmine has also shared the importance of her spiritual beliefs in helping her cope. Religion and spirituality can be protective factors for the development of psychological distress among Asian Americans (APA, 2012). The therapist in sessions explores ways Jasmine's spirituality has helped during this time by asking, "How does your temple and spirituality provide you support at this time?"

### Supporting Jasmine's Advocacy Needs

During the mid-phase of clinical treatment, Jasmine shares wanting to channel her anger and frustration constructively by exploring ways to take steps to advocate for her community. For example, by speaking up to her local elected board of supervisors to share her concerns on the recent increase in anti-Asian hate crimes in San Jose, California, she can practice self-empowerment in the face of societal marginalization. During the clinical sessions, the therapist helps Jasmine assess her readiness to speak out publicly in these ways. The therapist acknowledged Jasmine's stated vulnerability around this macrostep, so she helped her clarify the message she wished to send and determine whether sending it in an email would be an acceptable alternative. Such techniques provide agency and help empower Jasmine in feeling she is advocating in some way to support her community.

### Countertransference Considerations in This Case

Like with all clients, countertransference issues may arise for a therapist working with Jasmine. To best support Jasmine, as authors and therapists we explore the following countertransference issues that may arise and need to be addressed clinically to support Jasmine:

- The therapist may notice their own feelings get triggered in listening to Jasmine's experiences of racism, specifically around anti-Asian hate. If this is the case, it is helpful for the therapist to reflect on the feelings of overwhelm and assess whether these are detrimentally impacting the clinical work and if clinical consultation and supervision are needed.
- The therapist may have personal experiences of anti-Asian hate and racism, and working with Jasmine can create anger and frustration to arise for the therapist. If this is the case, the therapist should explore the countertransference, paying attention to whether the feelings are coming from their own anti-Asian hate experiences, and if so, to seek consultation and supervision to ensure it does not affect the clinical encounter.

As Asian American therapists, we reflect on the case of Jasmine and some of the countertransference we feel is the sadness and frustration of witnessing another Asian American female directly receive hate. Knowing this, if the authors were working with Jasmine, we would continue to ask open questions to remain curious about Jasmine's experiences. In sessions, if as therapists we felt anger or frustration, we would tap into these feelings and ground ourselves in the session and work to come back to tracking the client. Only if it feels clinically appropriate, as therapists we can also join and self-disclose that "As an Asian American, I also feel anger that this has happened to you" to help the client feel heard and validated. Finally, as authors working with Jasmine, we would continue to seek consultation and supervision to support Jasmine's needs.

## Relevance of Activism in Transformative Therapy

Therapists working with Asian American identified individuals like Jasmine should curiously consider the ways racial identity intersects with presenting problems such as anxiety and fear. Racism, racial identity, race-based stress, and religion and spirituality may be important topics to explore in clinical assessment, treatment planning, and interventions. In summary, engaging in transformative therapy as activism is about recognizing the intersection between mental health and societal issues clients encounter, such as racism and ways they can better support their clients clinically. The cost of not engaging in transformative therapy can be detrimental to clients like Jasmine, and therapists need to be aware of their own biases and engage in clinical support, consultation, and trainings. As therapists working with Asian American clients like Jasmine, the consequences of not engaging in therapy as activism can be significant and can include clients not receiving the support they need to address issues related to oppression, discrimination, and trauma. Therapists may inadvertently perpetuate harm or retraumatize clients through lack of understanding or insensitivity to the client's cultural needs. Both Asian American and non-Asian American identified therapists may need training on how to address race-based stressors and should seek materials that give tangible ideas for doing this work. Marriage and family therapists continue to engage in a lifelong journey of learning and advocacy to best support their clients.

## Reflection Questions

### Questions for the Therapist

- How do you define advocacy in therapy? What are your beliefs in advocacy for clients?
- How do you define activism?
- In what ways have your racial and cultural identity and personal experiences (such as family migration legacies, socioeconomic status) impacted how you engage in activism as a therapist?
- What supports may you need in creating transformative therapy spaces for your Asian American clients?

### Questions for Therapy

- How do you bring the topic of race and racial identity when the client does not bring it up as a presenting problem or concern?
- How do you understand advocacy and activism? How important are they to you? (to client)
- How have anti-Asian hate experiences impacted you and people you know? (to client)
- How do you cope with race-based stressors and racism? (to client)

## References

American Association for Marriage and Family Therapy. (2015). *AAMFT code of ethics*. AAMFT.

American Psychological Association. (2012). *Recommendations for the treatment of Asian-American/Pacific Islander populations*. https://www.apa.org/pi/oema/resources/ethnicity-health/asian-american/psychological-treatment

California Association for Marriage and Family Therapists. (2019). *CAMFT code of ethics*. CAMFT. https://www.camft.org/Membership/About-Us/Association-Documents/Code-of-Ethics

Cheng, H. L., Kim, H. Y., Reynolds (Taewon Choi), J. D., Tsong, Y., & Joel Wong, Y. (2021). COVID-19 anti-Asian racism: A tripartite model of collective psychosocial resilience. *American Psychologist, 76*(4), 627–642. https://doi.org/10.1037/amp0000808

Chopra, S. B. (2021). Healing from internalized racism for Asian Americans. *Professional Psychology: Research and Practice, 52*(5), 503–512. https://doi.org/10.1037/pro0000407

Dana, D. (2020). *Polyvagal exercises for safety and connection: 50 client-centered practices (Norton Series on Interpersonal Neurobiology)*. WW Norton & Company.

Delgado, R. & Stefancic, J. (2017). *Critical race theory* (3rd ed.). New York University Press. 10.18574/9781479851393

Duldulao, A. A., Takeuchi, D. T., & Hong, S. (2009). Correlates of suicidal behaviors among Asian Americans. *Archives of Suicide Research, 13*, 277–290.

Erolin, K. S., & Wieling, E. (2020). The experiences of couple/marriage and family therapists of color: A survey analysis. *Journal of Marital and Family Therapy, 47*(1), 3–20. https://doi.org/10.1111/jmft.12456

Franco, M., Durkee, M., & McElroy-Heltzel, S. (2021). Discrimination comes in layers: Dimensions of discrimination and mental health for multiracial people. *Cultural Diversity and Ethnic Minority Psychology, 27*(3), 343–353. https://doi.org/10.1037/cdp0000441

Fogelin, L. (2007). History, ethnography, and essentialism: The archaeology of religion and ritual in South Asia. *The Archaeology of Ritual, 3*, 23–42.

Hall, G. C. N., & Yee, A. (2012). U.S. mental health policy: Addressing the neglect of Asian Americans. *Asian American Journal of Psychology, 3*(3), 181–193. 10.1037/a0029950.

Helms, J. E. (1990). *Black and white racial identity: Theory, research, and practice*. Greenwood Press.

Holyoak, D., McPhee, D., Hall, G., & Fife, S. (2021). Microlevel advocacy: A common process in couple and family therapy. *Family Process, 60*(2), 654–669. https://doi.org/10.1111/famp.12620

Iftikar, J. S., & Museus, S. D. (2018). On the utility of Asian Critical (AsianCrit) Theory in the field of education. *International Journal of Qualitative Studies in Education, 31*(10), 935–949. https://doi.org/10.1080/09518398.2018.1522008

Ladson-Billings, G., & Tate, W. F. (1995). Toward a critical race theory of education. *Teachers College Record, 97*(1), 47–68. https://doi.org/10.1177/016146819509700104

Lee, S., & Waters, S. F. (2021). Asians and Asian Americans' experiences of racial discrimination during the COVID-19 pandemic: Impacts on health outcomes and the buffering role of social support. *Stigma and Health, 6*(1), 70–78. https://doi.org/10.1037/sah0000275

Menakem, R. (2017). *My grandmother's hands: racialized trauma and the pathway to mending our hearts and bodies*. Central Recovery Press.

Moodley, R., Mujtaba, F., & Kleiman, S. (2018). Critical race theory and mental health. In B. Cohen (Ed.) *Routledge international handbook of critical mental health* (1st ed.) (pp. 79–88). Routledge. https://doi.org/10.4324/9781315399584-11

Museus, S. D., & Iftikar, J. (2013). An Asian Critical Theory (AsianCrit) framework. In M. Y. Danico & J. G. Golson (Eds.), *Asian American students in higher education* (pp. 18–29). Routledge.

Moss, L. J., & Singh, A. A. (2015). White school counselors becoming racial justice allies to students of color: A call to the field of school counseling. *Journal of School Counseling, 13*(5), 2–36. https://files.eric.ed.gov/fulltext/EJ1062933.pdf

Nadal, K. L. (2018). *Microaggressions and traumatic stress.* American Psychological Association.

Nadal, K. L. (2019). The brown Asian American movement: Advocating for South Asian, Southeast Asian, and Filipino American communities. *Asian American Policy Review, 29*, 2–11, 95. https://aapr.hkspublications.org/2020/02/02/the-brown-asian -american-movement-advocating-for-south-asian-southeast-asian-and-filipino-ameri- can-communities/

Panchal, K., & Alif, A. (2023). Religion, spirituality, and clinical implications. In U. Thakore-Dunlap, D. Srivastava, & N. Tewari (Eds.), *Counseling and Psychother- apy for South Asian Americans* (pp. 127–143). Routledge. https://doi.org/10.4324 /9781003081548-8

Sharma, J. & Hipolito-Delgado, C. P. (2021). Promoting anti-racism and critical con- sciousness through a critical counseling theories course. *Teaching and Supervision in Counseling, 3*(2), 15–25. https://doi.org/10.7290/tsc030203

Singh, A. A., Appling, B., & Trepal, H. (2020). Using the multicultural social justice counseling competencies to decolonize counseling practice: The important roles of theory, power, and action. *Journal of Counseling & Development, 98*(3), 261–271. https://doi.org/10.1002/jcad.12321

Sue, D. W., & Sue, D. (1999). *Counseling the culturally different: Theory and practice* (3rd ed.). John Wiley & Sons.

Root, M. P. P. (1990). Resolving "other" status: Identity development of biracial indi- viduals. *Women & Therapy, 9*(1), 185. https://doi.org/10.1300/J015v09n01_11

Salahuddin, N. M., & O'Brien, K. M. (2011). Challenges and resilience in the lives of urban, multiracial adults: An instrument development study. *Journal of Counseling Psychology, 58*(4), 494–507. https://doi.org/10.1037/a0024633

Tatum, B. (2003). *"Why are all the black kids sitting together in the cafeteria?": And other conversations about race.* Basic Books.

Thakore-Dunlap, U., Srivastava, D., & Tewari, N. (Eds.) (2023). *Counseling and psycho- therapy for South Asian Americans: Identity, psychology, and clinical implications.* Routledge.

U.S. Census Bureau. (2018). Demographic turning points for the United States. Popu- lation projections from 2020 to 2060. https://www.census.gov/content/dam/Census/ library/publications/2018/demo/P25_1144.pdf

Van der Kolk, B. A. (2014). *The body keeps the score: Brain, mind, and body in the heal- ing of trauma.* Viking.

Watts-Jones, D. (2002). Healing internalized racism: The role of a within-group sanctu- ary among people of African descent. *Family Process, 41*(4), 591–601. https://doi.org /10.1111/j.1545 5300.2002.00591.x

Williams, M. T., Holmes, S., Zare, M., Haeny, A., & Faber, S. (2022a). An evidence- based approach for treating stress and trauma due to racism. *Cognitive and Behavioral Practice.* 30(4):565-588 https://doi.org/10.1016/j.cbpra.2022.07.001

Williams, T., Faber, S. C., & Duniya, C. (2022b). Being an anti-racist clinician. *Cognitive Behaviour Therapist, 15, e19.* https://doi.org/10.1017/S1754470X22000162

Yoo, H. C., Jackson, K. F., Guevarra, R. P., Miller, M. J., & Harrington, B. (2016). Construction and initial validation of the Multiracial Experiences Measure (MEM). *Journal of Counseling Psychology, 63*(2), 198–209. https://doi.org/10.1037/cou0000117

# Part III

# Transforming Our Inheritance

This body has been surveilled
since I was formed
in my Ammu's fetus
growing in my Nani's womb.
My ancestors sacrificed with indigo stained palms
because the colonizers of Calcutta couldn't tell
our brown skin apart–
our own skin watching us for them.
The 1853 fingerprint invention was the surveillance
of the jungles, the thugees, the coolies
with ancient tongues–
too complicated for the British
yet too easy to sign away land, people, lives
with just a print of the thumb.
The first time my Nani voted
in an election of a decolonized partitioned land
she came home elated with her fingertips stained blue.
She and all the Aunties placed their first vote
for a woman–
1965 South Asian Suffragists
their ink stained fingerprints as proof of their voice,
With my own hands I used to eat my
Nani's rolled rotis indented with her palm.
Her fingerprints had tales to tell–
arched imprints of escaped mutiny by train
whirled stories of being spied on
with an imprisoned husband
loops of narratives of struggle, survival.
Oh, the stories that our skin holds secret.
When I was finally born
halfway around the world,

DOI: 10.4324/9781003321590-10

my baby feet were dipped in ink.
My birth was certified and this body
surveilled from that very moment.
Even here, they watch our brown skin
Fear-mongered into a corner with
A target on our backs.
Fingerprints have turned into
countering violent extremism biometrics–
my voice is betrayed by Alexa
my face is followed by hidden cameras
where I move is tracked by apps on my phone.
They are surveilling it all, us all.
Ink-swirled by my ancestors
catch these hands.
Just like the motherland
we can decolonize these lands.
When I place my vote today with these fingers
I am channeling the ancestral yesteryears
that got us here.
I vote into the future
Because I know my ancestors of past
have placed their ink-stained palms on my back
in present.
Our own skin is watching us for them–
Nani's fingerprints embedded in mine.

Ahmed, T. (2020 October 27). *Catch these ink stained hands* [Video]. YouTube.
https://www.youtube.com/watch?v=_YBks7O-J_s&t=116s

# Chapter 7

# Constructing Shame Resilience as Asian Americans

## Face, Race, and Bicultural Identity

*Natalie Hsieh and Jessica ChenFeng*

The resurgence of anti-Asian racism, xenophobia, and hate crimes during the COVID-19 pandemic has made Asian American racial trauma and mental health needs more visible and palpable (Wu et al., 2021). However, Asian Americans are the least likely racial group to seek therapy, citing stigma, shame, and "loss of face" concerns as reasons to decline services (Masuda & Boone, 2011; SAMHSA, 2023). Furthermore, Asian Americans who do go to therapy feel less understood when therapists do not attune to their *relational* identity, which is shaped by collectivist, racialized, and bicultural experiences (ChenFeng et al., 2017). How can we guide therapy that helps Asian American clients feel more fully seen and supported in building shame resilience?

In this chapter, we highlight key features of Asian American lived experience so that clinicians can honor and support diverse expressions of Asian American identity resilience. Our clinical recommendations are grounded in self-reflection and findings from dissertation interviews that I (Natalie) conducted to explore themes of shame and shame resilience within the identity narratives of 1.5[1] and second-generation Chinese[2] Americans.[3] Through hearing participant stories, I became significantly more in touch with my racial identity journey. I had an "aha" moment when I realized the impact of internalized racism on the intergenerational disconnects and conflicts I ached to see bridged and healed in first and second-generation families and church families.

I (Jessica) served on Natalie's dissertation committee, and while I had spent many years working with Asian American clients, I found Natalie's research groundbreaking and extremely applicable for clinical practice. Even if not explicitly or consciously identified, the experience of shame seems to have a strong orienting force for the reason that Asian Americans seek therapy. Through the white gaze, there is a deep judgment and dismissal of the concept of shame—"What's wrong with Asian culture that it causes so many Asians/ Asian Americans to feel shame?" or "What's wrong with my parents/family?" The unfortunate but all too common clinical goal is to get clients to stop feeling shame without exploring the relational and structural layers of origin. This can add to the complex layers of internalized racism for Asian American clients.

DOI: 10.4324/9781003321590-11

This chapter centers our Asian American voice on understanding shame, and how honoring the witness of shame can be a powerful way to name and explore identity complexities and relational pain in therapy. From an individual Western lens, it is easy to characterize shame as a "negative" emotional trait, something to heal from and move beyond. When we center a relational "we" identity which is foundational to many Asian American contexts, we can better understand our clients' shame and support their identity resilience.

## Personal Connection to Topic (Natalie)

I (Natalie) am a cultural insider to my research, the younger of two daughters of parents from China and Hong Kong who came to the United States as students. I experience my Chinese cultural identity deepest through relationships with my parents and sister, my Taiwanese American spouse, and our extended families. I have also been shaped by my Chinese Christian "church families"—my "home" church where I developed lifelong friendships and met my spouse, and the Chinese and Taiwanese congregations my spouse has pastored in the last two decades. Being a daughter of church leaders and a pastor's spouse has shaped my sense of *face*—how my personal actions, example, and leadership connect to the well-being and representation of my family and community. My location within a millennial cohort of second-generation, Southern California Asian Americans also shapes my voice and vantage point on identity construction.

My interest in shame and shame resilience began decades ago when my college psychology major opened my access to a world of topics that felt new or taboo in my Chinese community: emotions, mental illness, trauma, abuse, and relational conflict. I was stunned that whole families could talk about shame-activating concerns in front of a professional. Intrigued to see if family therapy could disarm the power of shame, I trained with hopes of strengthening Asian American families and church families for greater intergenerational healing and flourishing. Since then, I have also become passionate about encouraging Asian American contributions to our field's understanding of family life expressions.

I felt excited when Brené Brown's public speaking and writing began making shame part of our everyday conversation. But while part of me resonated with Brown's shame resilience theory (2006), significant parts of me felt untouched. Like many theorists before her, Brown highlights shame as an *individual*'s internal negative experience and shame resilience as an individual's process of resolving shame. As a bicultural Chinese American, I experience shame largely as a *relational* emotion—disconnection or pain in relationships with family, cultural community, or society (Wong et al., 2014). I worry when an individual's agency or boundary-setting exacerbates loss of face for their family or increases guilt or strain for disrupting family/cultural norms. I wanted to construct a shame resilience theory that highlights *relational* shame, as well as the complicated process of constructing an internal sense of self while navigating multiple cultures.

My qualitative research was designed with therapy in mind. The interview guide explores identity stories conversationally, making it easier to attune to themes of relational attachment, shame, and resilience. Questions draw from an intergenerational and postmodern narrative understanding of identity, in which identity is socially located and constructed by personal and family history, roles and relationships, migration and racialization experiences, social discourses, and cultural norms.

## Personal Connection to Topic (Jessica)

As the elder of two, second-generation Taiwanese American daughters, being sensitive, aware, and responsive to the realities of shame and face was simply part of my existence. In my family, these were deeply intertwined with cultural values of honor and care for elders and Christian family values of giving and service. When my paternal grandmother was alive, my dad would visit her every day at her senior apartment home to spend time with her, bringing her the Chinese newspaper to read and eating together. This filial piety was part of the culture at church, where the "youth" (second-generation grandchildren) regularly served lunch first to our elders (grandparents) and were attentive to their needs. I can't speak for all the youth, but perhaps because of my parents' own positive relationships with their parents and modeling of filial piety, I found it enjoyable and meaningful to have relationships with the *ahmas (grandmas)* and *ahgongs (grandpas)* of my Taiwanese American immigrant church. In the social context of this immigrant church, there was an awareness that other parents and grandparents were observing and aware of the youth's degree of filial piety and honor of elders, and it was communally praised and valued. There was an implicit understanding that in being a caring and dutiful grandchild, your parents had raised you well.

Because of my role as the elder daughter (and the intersections of my personality mixed with family dynamics), I did not deviate from what was expected of me. In a way, you could say that I avoided feeling shame and was able to save face—really for my family and less so for myself.

There are countless daily relational encounters that shaped my consciousness around shame and face, and my relationship with these felt realities continues to shift as my bicultural and racial identity transforms over time and context. This is what I have also seen in the lives of Asian American clients. So much of "traditional therapy" training is inadequate in giving language to the nuanced and often unspoken relational emotions of collectivist family and community life. I am grateful that Natalie's research offers us some of this articulation which can serve to bring validation and healing to our communities.

## Theoretical and Conceptual Background

Shame is a universal human experience, but *culture* profoundly shapes its meaning (Goetz & Keltner, 2007; Wong & Tsai, 2007). In the United States, where

Western culture focuses on the *individual*, shame is described as an *individual*'s internal experience. Shame is considered maladaptive, interfering with cultural ideals of personal autonomy, agency, and self-worth (Erikson, 1980; Van Vliet, 2008; Brown, 2012) and contributing to poor psychological outcomes (Wong & Tsai, 2007). Many theorists contrast shame ("I *am* bad") with guilt ("I *did* something bad"), because shame often spirals into a totalizing negative view of self, whereas guilt can motivate a person to correct negative actions and make relational repairs (Brown, 2006; Wong & Tsai, 2007). From a Western cultural standpoint, shame resilience is an *individual*'s process of exercising agency to critically evaluate shame messaging, connect with others, and grow from shame (Brown, 2006; Van Vliet, 2008).

Asian American attunement to *relational identity* reframes shame in three significant ways. First, an Asian *collectivist* understanding of self challenges our assumption that shame is always maladaptive. In Asian communities, shame is an adaptive and essential marker of group standards, motivating members to align with elders, promote harmony, and represent one's family/group honorably (Wong et al., 2014; Greenber & Iwakabe, 2011). Shame, considered "losing face" for one's family/group, is experienced as isolation or exclusion, a threat to cultural ideals of group belonging and harmony (Wong & Tsai, 2007). Second, the *racialized* self of Asian Americans shows that shame is not only a "self-conscious" emotion (Tracy et al., 2007) but also a "socially conscious" one: Asian Americans' experiences as the unseen, othered, or excluded "model minority" and "forever foreigner" bear witness to their shamed position in the American racial hierarchy throughout their immigration history (Shih et al., 2019; Tuan, 1998). Third, the *bicultural* self of Asian Americans illuminates the complexity of managing public and private identities according to disparate social codes (Ting-Toomey, 2015), where shame can be internalized as disconnection from family or peers, or as ambiguous loss of belonging to either/both Asian heritage or American cultures (Benet-Martínez et al., 2002; Navarrete & Jenkins, 2011; Yeh & Hwang, 2000).

Our assumptions about identity and shame affect how we address shame in therapy. Therapists focusing on clients' *internal* shame may major in helping clients exercise personal agency to regulate emotions and enact boundaries to limit or opt out of challenging relationships. While helpful, this misses Asian Americans' collectivist, racialized, and bicultural layers of *relational* self, disrupting rapport or progress for some clients. By locating shame experiences within larger social and cultural contexts, we can enrich our clients' exploration of identity and empower culturally congruent visions of resilience.

## Experiences of Face, Race, and Bicultural Identity Shame

I (Natalie) once heard the word picture of a duck, smoothly swimming over tranquil waters yet paddling furiously under the surface, to describe hidden struggles of high-performing students. This metaphor is apt for bicultural Asian American experience as well. Asian Americans make many internal and relational identity negotiations and adjustments beneath the surface—at times consciously or strategically, yet often without full awareness or self-reflection.

In this section, we introduce *face*, *race*, and *bicultural* social "codebooks" of identity to organize and explore Asian American clients' "underwater" negotiation of identity across family/cultural and American/racial spaces. These codebooks help us notice how shame looks and feels and impacts identity attachment in each context. Figure 7.1 depicts how *face* shapes one's home identity within family/cultural relationships, *race* shapes identity within the broader "home" of American society, and how *bicultural identity* evolves dynamically as the intersection of these identities. This diagram reminds us that "Asian" and "American" cultural worlds are not equal and opposite; Asian American racial history influences how individual families and family members construct and manage their identities over time. Pseudonyms are used in the sharing of participant direct quotes, and clinical case examples reflect composite life experiences.

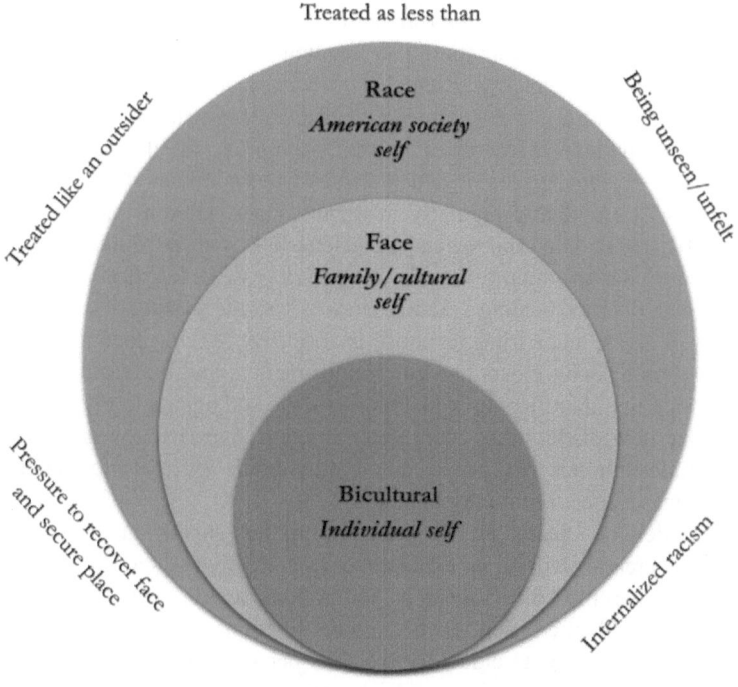

*Figure 7.1* Face, race, and bicultural identity layers of self (Hsieh, 2021)

## Face Identity Shame

> It's tough. 10 years ago I dropped out of college and I feel like from then until now I've always been trying to be successful… certain times when I would call my dad, it would make me sad that I'm not at the point in life where I can comfortably feel like, "Hey, I've made my dad proud."
>
> – *Michael, second-generation Chinese American*

For many Asian Americans, the *face* codebook operates at home, within one's Asian family/kin group or collective (e.g., neighborhood, friend network, church). My (Natalie's) participants described *face* as social currency that represents one's prestige or acceptability in one's family—where face can be saved, gained, or lost, depending on how one upholds family/group standards and fulfills expected social roles (e.g., eldest son, older sister, pastor/teacher). Face is more than one's physical appearance or social reputation; saving face reflects *relational* loyalty and a commitment to serve and honorably represent one's family.

Typically, Asian elders (e.g., parents, grandparents, appointed cultural or spiritual leaders) set group standards and norms, with mothers and older siblings cited as actively helping family members maintain face. While the priority of saving face may fade for nuclear families without strong connections to extended family or Asian community, it is often amplified when they do. Growing up, I (Natalie) called my parents' friends from our Chinese Christian church "aunties" and "uncles," and formed deep friendships with my same-generation peers. Our parents cared for each other's children and elders, labored in love to serve our church family, and welcomed international students and new immigrants. We gathered regularly in homes and at church for worship services, spiritual education, and special occasions like weddings, memorials, and baptisms. Regular community advice was abuzz (e.g., best grocery stores, Asian restaurants, doctors, healing practitioners), as was the sharing of social or professional resources, and caring for those in need. By "saving face" for my community—aligning with elders and community beliefs and practices, I was tacitly reaffirming my identification and honor to serve and belong to my group. I did not realize how distinct this "family-community" experience was until I visited non-ethnic churches that focused on an individual's spiritual experience, without expecting deeper community belonging.

The *face* codebook challenges the assumption that shame can be fully described as an internal, individual experience. In collectivist contexts, shame describes cut-off or ruptured relationships and is considered "losing face" for one's family/group. Shame is felt when one fails to fulfill social roles or cultural expectations, disappoints elders, or exposes personal/family weaknesses that cause others to lose trust in, pity, or talk negatively about one's family in the community. Shame can also be felt vicariously, through holding in a family secret or carrying unprocessed or unresolved grief. Because of the interconnectedness of individual/group identity, shame need not be verbalized to be implicitly felt when within a group (Wong et al., 2014). As such, it is not uncommon for Asian Americans to keep in their emotional burdens from trauma, grief, relational conflict, or to quietly withdraw from their community when they act or feel out of alignment, in order not to burden others, or because the pain or fear of losing face is too heavy.

*Face* identity shame can also affect a client's access and progress in therapy. The act of disclosing personal or family struggles, or talking about private emotional topics with someone "outside the family" (e.g., a therapist) can activate a sense of "losing face" for the family. It is also not uncommon for Asian Americans to refrain from letting a therapist know when they feel "missed" or misunderstood, out of a desire to not embarrass the therapist or cause the therapist to "lose face." This can pose challenges for building deeper therapeutic rapport and progress.

Examples of clinical concerns that connect to face-based shame include the following:

- **Treated like an outsider in one's family/community:** Gary, an associate pastor in an Asian immigrant church, was let go after taking a more progressive stance on a social issue, which church elders and senior leadership felt could sow discord and threaten church unity and trust. He is experiencing depression and identity/existential crisis, as he has lost face in a community he had invested in for over a decade like his family.
- **Treated as less than in one's family/community:** Susan feels disempowered and criticized by her family for not fulfilling cultural expectations for getting married and bearing children. As the youngest daughter in her family, Susan internalized that she doesn't know enough, isn't responsible, and must defer to elders and males. To avoid constantly being discussed among her family friend network, Susan moved far away to start afresh. She is feeling lonely and guilty for her choices and feels conflicted about how to return home when she finds out that her dad has cancer.
- **Being unseen or unfelt:** Jen feels she could never share her social and emotional world with her parents, who worked multiple jobs and were task-oriented, focusing on her studies and achievements. Jen felt lonely and isolated, despite becoming outwardly academically successful. In college, Jen plunged into romantic relationships in secret because she knew her parents would not approve. When her partner began showing signs of intimate partner violence, Jen felt fearful and depressed but unable to turn to anyone.

### Race Identity Shame

*Third grade is probably the earliest that I can remember, in terms of experiencing... that cultural difference, where I went from being super excited that*

> *I had noodles and kimchi packed for lunch, to being so incredibly embar-*
> *rassed, and upset that I had noodles and kimchi for lunch...This is when my*
> *story starts of me wanting to become more and more white.*
> *– Daniel, second-generation Taiwanese American*

Many Asian Americans socialize into their racial identity while navigating rela-tionships "outside" of home, such as in school, work, clubs, teams, or neighbor-hood spaces. However, some ideas about race are formed at home: it is common for immigrant families to say "white" or "Western" as a proxy for "American" (Tran & Paterson, 2016) or to use terms like "Westernized or "whitewashed" to describe the adopting of white-normed standards (e.g., playing certain sports, style of dress or music, chosen peers or partners, level of independence or self-expression). At times, Asian immigrant families also circulate ideas about how they compare to other Asian immigrants or other ethnic/racial groups in America. There is diversity in how Asian American families integrate relation-ally within broader American society—some immerse into immigrant/refugee or ethnic-specific neighborhoods, others engage regularly outside of the Asian community in school, work, or business, and still others intentionally choose diverse relationships, group affiliations, and life philosophies.

The *Race* codebook challenges the assumption that shame is primarily an internal emotion to regulate, illuminating collective shame experienced by immigrants/refugees and racial minorities within a larger social hierarchy. It surprised me (Natalie) how many participants shared a race-based shame expe-rience when I asked them: "When or how did you first become conscious of being Chinese American?" Many described moments when they felt invisible, othered, excluded, exoticized, or put down by peers or colleagues in connection to their Asianness (e.g., physical appearance, language ability, foods, ability or achievements, social mannerisms, temperament) or immigration status (e.g., new immigrant, refugee). Their everyday experiences also mirrored Asian American stereotypes of being unseen on the continuum of the white and Black binary, or perceived as the "forever foreigner" or "model minority" in American society (Shih et al., 2019; Tuan, 1998). Additionally, in conducting interviews during the COVID-19 pandemic, I engaged in frequent conversations about the viscer-ally felt resurgence of "yellow peril" racial slurs and violence toward Asians in America (Wu et al., 2021).

Consciousness of racial identity shame can shape everyday ways we carry ourselves in the world. When I (Jessica) was a doctoral student, I remember crossing a crosswalk with one of my white classmates. It was a four-way stop, so there were cars on every side waiting for us to walk across the street. As we started walking, I was rushing across while my friend seemed to take their time. What we discovered is that my friend was functioning under the idea of "we're the pedestrians so we have the right of way" whereas I was unconsciously trying to avoid collective racial shame because if I moved too slow, what would all these drivers think about Asian Americans! There was a racialized cost if I wasn't experienced as thoughtful of the drivers waiting for me to cross the street. It was not about me, but the racial group I represented.

Race-based shame can also impact the course of therapy, or of becoming a therapist. I (Natalie) remember feeling like an outsider to the field of therapy as a student, both because of the felt cultural incongruence of speaking openly about private emotional topics, and the fact that experts we read or watched did not often understand family dynamics in ways that resembled mine. I also remember the subtle cues of othering when Asian Americans and other people of color became topics of study as "other families" or "diverse families." While training and as a therapy client with non-Asian therapists, I often unconsciously carried the burden of whether I was sufficiently matching the expected "emotion language" or speaking "openly and directly enough" to feel seen and under-stood—the same racial burdens I carried in my everyday life.

Examples of clinical concerns that connect to race-based shame include the following:

- **Treated like an outsider in society:** David feels othered by peers showing disgust for Asian foods, and like a misfit without participation in "American" pastimes (e.g., camping, football). He copes with stress by generally being on his own, or by doing his work and not drawing attention to himself. Today in his marriage, his spouse complains that his passivity and difficulty with intimacy are putting a strain on their relationship.
- **Treated as less than in society:** Daniel reflects on a childhood full of teas-ing for his eye shape, spoken language, skin color—anything that overtly communicated his Asianness. This led to internalized shame, self-rejection, and self-loathing, including a season of regular suicidal ideation, distancing from Asian peers, and family conflict.
- **Being unseen or unfelt:** Alice grew up feeling culturally unseen and super-ficially known as a Taiwanese American ("Is Taiwan a country? Is that Thailand?"). She also reflects on how Asians are perceived safe and timid, expected to "keep quiet" in social settings. She realizes this contributes to her struggle to speak up in workplace settings, or to ask for what she wants or needs with friends or a romantic partner.

### Bicultural Identity Shame

*And then I think, as I mentioned, during middle school and high school there was this inner conflict where, I wouldn't say it was a hostile feeling, but I wasn't proud of being Chinese. It was really difficult speaking to my mom about it too, because she would always be like, "[Ellen], you have to do A, B, C, D, because it's Chinese heritage," and I'm like, "No, I'm American. Why couldn't we have been white?"*

*— Ellen, second-generation Chinese American*

The *bicultural* identity journeys of Asian Americans help us not take for granted that one moves in society with a singular or cohesive identity. Asian American immigrant families offer a window into the collision of "old and new worlds," and how losses, pressures, hopes, and role shifts can stretch and strain family relationships and worldviews (ChenFeng et al., 2015). It is not uncommon for family members to construct bicultural identity and experience shame very differently. First- or 1.5-generation Asian/Asian Americans grounded in face identity may encode racism during migration as a necessary rite of passage, sacrificing self to secure their family's future through education, economic stability, and marriage/childrearing. To regain face and home is to nurture relationships in Asian community, honor elders, and secure their children's future. Second-generation Asian Americans often more actively wrestle with, negotiate, and experiment with their internal "Asian identity" and "American identity," wondering where and with whom they best fit or feel at home. Race-based shame can evoke questions about whether it is safe or beneficial to embrace the cultural home of their parents or to show an Asian "face" in society. Furthermore, encounters with American discourse on race may provoke greater self-reflection on racial justice, equity, and representation of Asian Americans.

Bicultural identity shame, internalized at the crossroads of being Asian in American society, was described in three main ways. Many 1.5-generation participants described their *family's loss of face* from social/economic upheaval during migration, which motivated an anxious plunging of self into language, culture, and professional learning to recover family face and establish security. Others described their internal sense of *disconnection* and *isolation*—"not belonging anywhere" and not feeling "Asian enough" or "American enough" to feel at home in either space. Still others related the pain of *internalized racism*—experiences of race-based shame that led them to encode Asianness as inferior to whiteness—which at times resulted in deep self-rejection and relational conflict, resentment, or distancing from Asian family members, peers, and communities. At times, active hiding or suppression of one's Asian ethnic/racial identity—especially during the rise of Asian hate in the COVID-19 pandemic—became a matter of physical as well as psychological safety.

Examples of clinical concerns that connect to bicultural identity shame include the following:

- **Pressure to recover face and secure place:** John is having severe backaches and is feeling depressed and unmotivated since completing his graduate degree and beginning his full-time job. Now that life has slowed down,

John's body and mind may finally be registering the weight of the years he spent in "survival mode," suppressing his needs in order to hurry up and learn English, graduate with honors, and secure a prestigious job—all to make his parents' sacrifices for the family worth it.

- **Not belonging anywhere:** Rose feels profound loss of home country, neighborhoods, and extended family during migration, intensified by news of the loss of her beloved grandmother after arriving in the United States. She pushes through her losses and anxiety over not fitting in with American students by trying to learn English quickly, talking and dressing like others, and working extra hard to quiet her feelings of grief.

- **Internalized racism:** Lily gets into heated conflicts with her parents over her slipping grades and distances herself from family and Asian church gatherings. Her parents feel disrespected and criticize her lack of family/church commitment. Lily shares that she started to feel embarrassed around white peers who either made fun of or exoticized her Asian facial features, which grew into a hostile, resentful feeling toward being Asian. Her active refusal to "fulfill an Asian stereotype" contributes to her conflict with her parents for their "Asian" ways, and her attempts to cut ties with her cultural community.

## Change Processes to Build Shame Resilience

*I've learned that emotional vulnerability with people that you know well and trust is the game changer...A lot of times people paint resilience to be this like, "Oh, you need to be strong. You need to fight back." But what I am learning in this season is that resilience looks like being honest with your-self and saying, "I need help." Or, "I can't do this on my own"... Or like, "I'm confused about my ethnic identity and I'd like to explore it further." I think, just saying that, shows more courage and resilience.*

*– Susan, second-generation Taiwanese American*

I (Natalie) appreciate how attachment-based therapy approaches speak to Asian Americans' longing for *home*—a secure relational and cultural base to nurture growth and flourishing. In this framework, shame signals *insecure* cultural attachment due to relational loss, disconnection, conflict, or pain. If shame is regularly experienced, internalized shame can lead to shame-based coping for social survival (e.g., deferring, hiding, suppressing, or cutting off/rejecting parts of oneself or cultural community). While shame-based coping can motivate hard work and resilience and even be necessary to achieve temporal security, it taxes mental, physical, and relational health over time. When an attachment-based therapy process is applied to shame and identity resilience, a therapist's primary clinical aims are:

(1) to help clients explore bicultural identity complexities and affirm their need for feeling at home within themselves (attachment need)
(2) to compassionately accept previously unseen/disowned parts of self, and to safely hold client experiences of relational distress and trauma (cultural/racial attachment shame)
(3) to encourage healing and growth through identity grounding and experiencing relational shame counterstories (cultural reconnection)
(4) to explore creative ways to envision and express whole-self resilience in various contexts (bicultural identity attachment)

We can glean clinically relevant insights from participants who shared how they moved from shame-based coping toward *whole-self resilience*, which involves exploring and expressing both Asian/ethnic and American social identities. Turning points involved *identity grounding* through greater consciousness and engagement with cultural/racial identity roots and history, and *relational shame counterstories*, where connection or acceptance is experienced in place of previous shame.

Participants found deeper *family/cultural* identity grounding through family and personal odysseys to countries of origin, conversation around family migration or resilience stories, or deeper learning of Asian languages, history, and cultural practices. They found deeper *racial* identity grounding by connecting personal/family struggles to a larger story arc of Asian American collective struggles and resilience, alongside histories of other immigrant groups and persons of color. They also experienced greater *bicultural* identity grounding upon "leaving home" (e.g., migration, leaving home for college, traveling outside the United States) and finding space to discover personal core values away from typical social scripts and settings.

Relational shame counterstories also mapped to family/cultural, racial, and bicultural identity contexts. Participants experienced relational repair from conflict or cultural clash with parents through caring for their parents or experiencing a more humanizing, empathetic relationship with them. Others described how guidance, advocacy, and mentorship from Asian Americans ahead of them helped them feel seen and more resourced when navigating the culture of school and work. Participants also described healing through "me too" moments and belonging with other "outsiders"—whether that be other Asian Americans, immigrants, or persons of color.

There is no one-size-fits-all vision for resilience (see Figure 7.2). Many shared changes in how they related to social groups. Some grew in solidarity with their family/cultural resilience stories, or promoted Asian/Asian American representation in society. Others became energized to interrupt racism by speaking up against injustice or standing with other persons of color, immigrants, or marginalized groups. Some exercised resilience as the "both/and" posture of code-switching (e.g., exercising flexibility of self to show deference to elders, then adjusting to more direct or casual communication style with others) or

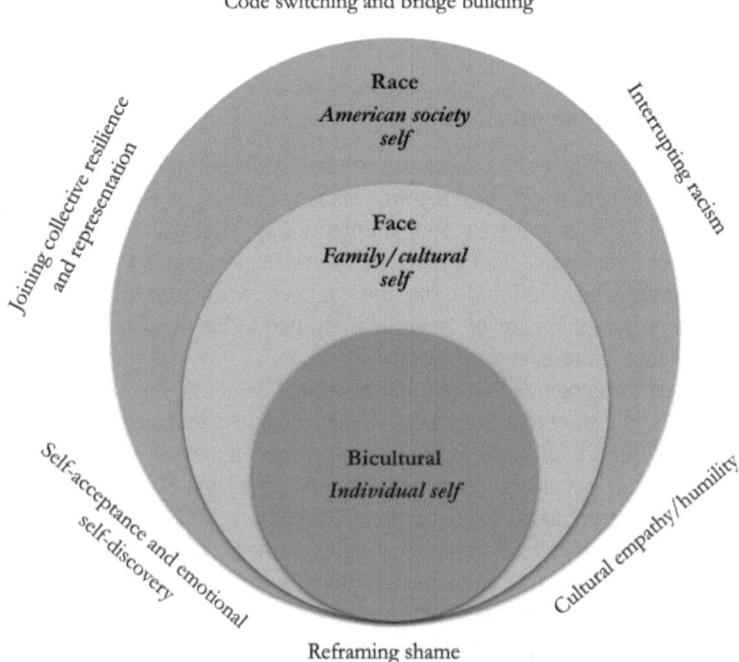

*Figure 7.2* Expressions of whole-self resilience (Hsieh, 2021)

bridge-building (e.g., offering instruction or correction about Asian American experiences in non-Asian spaces).

Participants' identity resilience was also marked by significant internal change through nurturing emotional attunement, individual self-discovery, and self-acceptance. Some generated a new vision of bicultural identity as the creative potential to be a "global citizen" who embodies "both/and" living. Participants also shared counterstories that reframed shame itself: some found a decisive spiritual identity home with God and Christian community, where divine love and community acceptance disarmed their fear of shame. Others found mentors and therapists who reframed the shame of emotional vulnerability or failure as opportunities to unpack emotional burdens and grow in self-compassion, courage, and humility.

## Clinical Recommendations

The therapist's role in building a secure attachment base for clients to explore identity and whole-self resilience in therapy is significant. We offer some clinical recommendations based on this research and lived experience within our

Asian American families and communities. These are certainly not exhaustive, but perhaps potentially helpful for framing ways to move toward the heart of addressing and inviting healing related to shame, face, and bicultural identity.

### Orient to Relational Identity

We have heard Asian American clients share that they discontinued therapy with therapists who missed or minimized the importance of joining with clients' "we" relational identity. This miss can happen unintentionally, through focusing only on a client's individual needs and concerns, by privileging client's self-expression without processing relational costs and changes expected with significant relationship/roles they carry, or by being less attuned to how therapist position and power impact the therapeutic relationship.

It is important to recognize that the first relational context being navigated in the room is with you, the therapist. Many clients consider the therapist to be the host and authority figure in the room, and out of respect may wait for a therapist to guide norms and expectations for the goals of therapy, level of self-disclosure, appropriate kinds of responses, and pace of conversation. I (Natalie) often have an explicit conversation with clients about the relational role and norms I envision for the therapy room (e.g., my role and style/approach, and my invitation for the client's role/expertise, etc.) and invite clients to share their comfort level with therapy and how well it fits with the way they have grown up communicating with others.

It is also important to get a sense of clients' relational orientation to self, family, other Asian Americans, other people of color, and to whiteness. Even if we are Asian American therapists, we cannot assume that our Asian American clients share similar ways of connecting across these relational spheres. During initial assessment, we can invite clients to share what cultural/racial identity they prefer to use (e.g., Korean American, Asian American, Asian), and to share about "important people and places outside of this room" including relationships with extended family, cultural/spiritual communities, cities or places they have lived or have family connections). We might also ask clients whether they identify as a certain generation, to glean how recent family migration was, and what identity reference points they have.

To be sensitive to the concerns about speaking "badly or negatively" about family members, I (Jessica) might preface my questions with something to the effect of:

> I want you to know that as I ask questions about your relationship with your parents, I know they did their best to raise you and that I hold deep respect for who they are and the many sacrifices they have made. I can imagine it's hard to say anything negative about them because it feels dishonoring. Even in our parents' best abilities, it's possible that there were unintended

consequences that we felt hurt or harmed by. I can see that both could be true at the same time.

This gives clients permission to more openly share what would typically be experienced as shameful (to the family) conversations because they can trust that the therapist is not judging their family or parents. It is important for the therapist within the therapeutic relationship to hold together with the client the significance and weight of this family and relational orientation and allows the client to feel that trust can be built.

I also want to mention to non-Asian therapists that there are ways you can further exacerbate racial shame and loss of face in the therapeutic space. Regardless of your racial consciousness and cultural humility/competence, Asian American clients come to therapy with their own (often unconscious) internalized racial stress and experiences with various racial groups. There is a racial relational reality in the therapeutic relationship that the therapist can speak to, if it seems clinically appropriate. For example, "It is different for every client, but sometimes conversation about race can be uncomfortable, awkward or painful. I want to let you know that I welcome these conversations. Is it okay if I check in with you about what it feels like to work with me, a _____ (therapist's racial or ethnic identity) therapist?" or "I'm generally aware of the complex ways that Asian Americans experience their racial identity and am committed to these conversations if they're important to you." It goes without saying that a therapist needs to be very aware of their own implicit biases related to Asian Americans so that these are not harmfully played out in clinical work.

### Invite Face, Race, and Bicultural Identity Stories into the Room

We believe there is a critical role that therapists play in inviting conversations about face, race, and identity into the room. It is more likely than not that our clients are consciously or unconsciously sensing if we are comfortable and able to have such conversations. They may also not be aware of the ways that issues of face, race, and identity shape their relational lives. We can thoughtfully assess how clients relate to face and race through inviting such stories.

We can identify stories of *face* through emotions related to a client's relational orientation toward self and family. There might be emotions of shame, guilt, worry, distress, or fear regarding something that the client has done, their concern for their family/ancestors, and how parents or others might be thinking of them. Conversely, there can be feelings of pride, excitement, relief, hope, or joy because of an experience of accomplishment and how this affects sense of self and relationship to family, parents, or the ethnic/racial group the client identifies with. Here are some possible ways to explore these stories:

- I see that this experience is stirring up some deep emotion for you. Can you tell me more about what it brings up for you? Is there someone you are holding close to you as you feel this way?
- What are some expectations you grew up with in your family? How did you become aware of those expectations? What would it have meant to align with the expectations or to distance from them?
- Do you remember some early experiences around how you learned to orient to yourself and others with this awareness?
- In what spaces or relationships do these feelings and thoughts most often show up?

Additionally, assessment tools such as the Brief Collectivism Questionnaire (Lui & Rollock, 2018) or the Asian American Values Scale (Kim, Ki, & Ng, 2005) can serve as a springboard for more conversations related to *face*. Therapists can also facilitate genogram work to understand the varying levels of connection to collectivist and relational identity of different family members to support the client in developing awareness about these often unspoken interconnections.

Each person, even within families, has a different way of understanding self as it relates to other Asian Americans, other people of color, and to whiteness. Clinicians can keep this in mind while tuning into clients' stories about *race*. These are possible ways of increasing consciousness about a client's relational identity as it relates to race:

- I would love to hear more about how you became aware of your racial/ethnic identity and what meaning that had/has for you.
- How is your relationship with being Asian American similar or different from that of your family members (or specifically spouse/partner, children, parents, etc.)?
- Did you grow up with a sense that being Asian American was different from being another racial identity? How so? In what ways and through whom did those messages show up?

Bicultural or multicultural identity can come with a range of weighty and complex experiences. Here are some ways to invite these stories into the room:

- How did you learn to navigate being both Asian (or specific ethnic identity) and "American" in the various parts of your life?
- Are there ways in which part(s) of your identity feel challenging to navigate? Have there been significant moments when you encountered this?
- How has your bicultural identity served you in life? Sources of pain? Sources of resilience?

### Honor the Witness of Relational Shame

The experience of shame is often an isolating experience and so the honoring and witnessing of it can be so powerfully healing. For all the complex reasons related to migration, cultural and generational disconnect, and language barriers, processing shame is not something that children learn to do with their parents. While shame is such a profound relational construct, it is rarely explicitly discussed or worked through in actual relationships. Thus the impact of intentional, delicate care that a therapist can offer in inviting and being present with these stories cannot be underestimated. Here are some possible ways to validate, reflect, value, affirm, and honor the client's process:

- I am struck by the courage (strength, resilience, etc.) it takes for you to speak this out loud.
- I can sense the weight of this, and it is an honor for me to bear this with you.
- I find myself impacted by your family's and your resilience in spite of...
- I do not take for granted how hard it is for you to share this with me. You are so brave.

With clinical discretion, self-disclosure (for Asian American therapists) or relating of themes from Figure 7.1 as experiences shared by many Asian Americans (e.g., "what you share sounds like it could connect with the experience of being unseen or like an outsider that many Asian Americans can relate to") can invite clients to feel greater normalization of their emotions and solidarity.

### Encourage Identity Grounding and Whole-Self Resilience

The path toward developing whole-self resilience has everything to do with clients reclaiming and re-envisioning their relationships with self across racial, ethnic, familial/cultural identities. Therapists can encourage this by supporting clients in their development of *contextual differentiation* (ChenFeng, 2018). This is increased through the process of becoming conscious of, identifying, and understanding personal thoughts and feelings as they are influenced by, related to, and different from one's context. In regard to face, shame, and bicultural identity, context can be embedded in family, ethnicity/culture, racial/larger U.S. society, and history.

It is not uncommon for Asian Americans to be disconnected from their family, ethnic, and racial histories because trauma kept the stories silent, or they were not written into textbooks or taught in U.S. history classes. While these histories include much loss, grief, and trauma, the cut-off from these stories also means cut-off from legacies of resilience and strength. Therapists can help clients in discovering and reconnecting with these stories:

- What do you know about your family's migration story? Might there be a relative that you can connect with to learn more about it?
- What stories do you remember hearing about your _____ (parents, grand-parents, aunts/uncles, etc.)? What do these stories tell you about your family?
- Asian American history is often left out of U.S. history or misrepresented. What is your understanding of and exposure to Asian American history? What do you know about _____ (client's ethnic identity/ies) American history? (There are a number of excellent resources on Asian American history. Please see list at the end of chapter)
- (if client has done some exploration and learning into Asian American history) How is what you are learning shaping and shifting your understanding of Asian Americans?

As clients move from disconnect and cut-off to curiosity and reconnection, they increase their capacity for whole-self resilience. Cut-off (from identity, stories, histories, relationships) has served a purpose, and identity grounding happens through the expansion of a both/and identity: that it is possible to have the legacy of generational trauma and legacy of resilience; that there are spaces where feeling racialized invisibility can happen and spaces where strength, voice, and empowerment can be activated. Understanding and identifying the how and why of these experiences increases contextual differentiation, expanding whole-self resilience and diffusing the crippling power of shame.

## Putting It All Together: Clinical Case Example

Ann, a 19-year-old Asian American female client is referred to therapy by her college roommate for symptoms of depression and self-harm after being sexually assaulted by her white boyfriend. If we only attune to Ann's individual and specific episode of trauma, we might encourage Ann to name and challenge shame fueling her negative self-view, offer tools for grounding and quieting traumatic stress, encourage connection with other survivors, and build resilience with self-affirmations. While this treatment focus would offer help and healing for Ann's individual and immediate symptoms, it would not touch the larger relational and cultural layers of trauma and shame. When a therapist invites Ann's personal and family identity stories and helps her attune to shame, this is an important part of self-validation and healing.

*Orient to relational identity.* As the therapist invites Ann's family and life stories into the room, it becomes clear that Ann's most immediately felt anxiety is in her perceived loss of face in violating the expectations of her family and spiritual community regarding sexual purity, and for her discussing private problems outside the family. Rather than dismissing parental or cultural expectations, the therapist names and normalizes Ann's fear of losing face for her family, affirms the importance of Ann's family and cultural relationships, and underlines a commitment to confidentiality in therapy. This allows her to release some of the distress around therapy potentially violating her personal, cultural, and familial values. She can consequently experience herself and understand her family and cultural experiences more fully and presently.

*Invite face, race, and bicultural identity stories.* In asking Ann about her family and cultural stories, she describes how her place as the only daughter in a fairly traditional and conservative Christian family meant very rigid assumptions and expectations about behavior and relationships. Articulating out loud the unspoken and spoken expectations of her upbringing helps Ann to recognize the pressure she had internalized and how this shapes the shame she feels. The therapist learns that Ann grew up and lives in a predominantly white community and the racism and financial stress her parents experienced in running a local Chinese restaurant fueled her desire to do everything right so she would not have to add to her parents' stress. She had few friends at school and at church that she could share these stories with.

*Honor the witness of relational shame.* As Ann develops greater trust in the therapeutic relationship, the therapist can invite her to explore how immediate trauma connects to larger stories of pain or disconnection. She explores how her current sense of emotional unsafety and emptiness first began when she felt emotionally unseen within her family, put on a pedestal by friends for her high academic achievement, and othered or exoticized for her Asian features by non-Asian peers in middle and high school. Ann starts to connect how her experience of sexual assault crystallized a core internal narrative of emotional placelessness, in that her attempts to escape loneliness by gaining white male acceptance still left her trapped and dishonored as an Asian American female. While these begin as cognitive conversations, they uncover a heavy and palpable embodied felt shame. Across sessions, there are moments where the shame has no words and the therapist postures herself with empathy and validation, showing Ann that she is not alone and is not being judged. By validating and creating safety for Ann to put words to layers of her contextual self, Ann's therapist helps Ann feel more grounded to explore the multiple meanings around shame and trauma.

*Encourage identity grounding and whole-self resilience.* The work of increasing contextual differentiation is already happening through Ann exploring stories of face, shame, and bicultural identity. It continues as the therapist asks Ann about her family's migration story and if she is learning about Asian American history in school. Ann returns a few weeks later energized by what she learned regarding her family's history. She did not know that her maternal grandfather was a freedom swimmer (escaped the communism of China for freedom in Hong Kong) and this reshaped the sense she was making about her family. Her mother shared about the expectations she experienced as a result of the significant risk and sacrifices grandfather had made. Ann started to understand the implicit expectations as her family's way of protecting, loving, and seeking survival in new and foreign places. This led to Ann being curious about Chinese American history, and the stories of resilience, especially with Chinese American women, allowed her to imagine her own voice becoming as powerful too, one day.

## Conclusion: Asian American Contributions to Shame Resilience

Asian American lives and stories contribute much to our conversation on identity and shame resilience. We are reminded that our identities are interconnected and dynamically shaped within relational and cultural contexts. As we invite bicultural identity stories into the room, we offer clients a secure relational base to feel more seen and known in their relational world. By honoring shame as a witness to cultural attachment insecurity, relational loss, and trauma, we can explore clinical concerns associated with internalized shame or shame-based coping with greater compassion and understanding. Our therapeutic process may invite clients to change through deeper identity grounding in family roots and collective Asian American history, and through a rich array of relational shame counterstories—humanizing family relationships, voicing pain and advocacy for justice, reframing "outsider" status to leader in both/and thinking and relating—and the precious gift of growing more at home embodying their whole selves.

## Reflection Questions

### Questions for the Therapist

- What is the experience of and role of shame in your own life? Through what contextual avenues was this shaped?
- How has this chapter uncovered some implicit biases you might have held about shame being a personal/individual experience vs a relational/contextual one?
- How has this chapter helped you consider new ways to attune to *relational identity*—the impact of relationships, group affiliations, and social codes and norms on the way personal identity is shaped and constructed?
- What are your portraits of what resilience looks like? How has this chapter reaffirmed or offered you new ideas for what resilience could look like for clients?

### Questions for Therapy (see chapter for additional questions)

- ***Relational Identity***: How connected do you feel to Asian culture? To American culture? (Any other cultures?) What relationships have helped you nurture these connections? What cultural identity label do you prefer to use?

- *Face*: What are some expectations you grew up with in your family of origin? How did you become aware of those expectations? What would it have meant to align with the expectations or to distance from them? How important is "saving face" in your family?
- *Race*: I'd love to hear more about how you became aware of your racial/ethnic identity and what meaning that had/has for you. How is your relationship with being Asian American similar or different from that of your family members (or specifically spouse/partner, children, parents, etc.)?
- *Bicultural identity*: How did you learn to navigate being both Asian (or specific ethnic identity) and "American" in the various parts of your life? When has this journey been difficult or painful? When have you experienced strength or resilience?

## Resources on Asian American History

- Lee, E. (2016). *The making of Asian America: A history*. First Simon & Schuster trade paperback edition. Simon & Schuster Paperbacks.
- https://asianamericanedu.org/
- https://www.naseemrdz.com/resources/asian-american-history-curriculum/

## Notes

1  1.5 generation refers to individuals who immigrated between the ages of 6 and 18 (Benyamin, 2018).
2  While this study recruited participants who identified as "Chinese American," participants also identified more specifically as Taiwanese American, Hong Kong American, and the integration of Chinese with Cambodian, Vietnamese, and Malaysian cultures.
3  For more information about study background, design, and findings, see Hsieh, N. (2021). Constructing Bicultural Identity and Shame Resilience in Chinese Americans (Doctoral dissertation, Loma Linda University).

## References

Benet-Martínez, V., Leu, J., Lee, F., & Morris, M. W. (2002). Negotiating biculturalism: Cultural frame switching in biculturals with oppositional versus compatible cultural identities. *Journal of Cross-Cultural Psychology, 33*(5), 492–516. https://doi.org/10.1177/0022022102033005005

Benyamin, N. A. (2018). The ethnic identity journey of 1.5 generation Asian American college students. University of Northern Colorado. *Dissertations*. 477. https://digscholarship.unco.edu/dissertations/477

Brown, B. (2006). Shame resilience theory: A grounded theory study on women and shame. *Families in Society, 87*(1), 43–52. https://doi.org/10.1606/1044 3894.3483

Brown, B. (2012). *Daring greatly: How the courage to be vulnerable transforms the way we live, love, parent, and lead*. Penguin.

ChenFeng, J. (2018). Integration of self and family: Asian American Christians in the midst of white Evangelicalism and being the model minority. In E. E. Wilson & L. Nice (Eds.), *Socially just religious and spiritual interventions: Ethical uses of therapeutic power.* Springer, 15-25.

ChenFeng, J., Kim, L., Wu, Y., & Knudson-Martin, C. (2017). Addressing culture, gender, and power with Asian American couples: Application of socio-emotional relationship therapy. *Family Process, 56*(3), 558–573. https://doi.org/10.1111/famp.12251

ChenFeng, J., Knudson-Martin, C., & Nelson, T. (2015). Intergenerational tension, connectedness, and separateness in the lived experience of first and second-generation Chinese American Christians. *Contemporary Family Therapy, 37*(2), 153–164. https://doi.org/10.1007/s10591-015-9335-9

Erikson, E. H. (1980). *Identity and the life cycle.* W.W. Norton & Company.

Goetz, J. L., & Keltner, D. (2007). Shifting meanings of self-conscious emotions across cultures: A social-functional approach. In J. L. Tracy, R. W. Robins, & J. P. Tangney (Eds.). *The self-conscious emotions: Theory and research* (pp. 153–173). The Guilford Press.

Greenberg, L., & Iwakabe, S. (2011). Emotion-focused therapy and shame. In R. L. Dearing & J. P. E. Tangney (Eds.). *Shame in the therapy hour* (pp. 69–90). American Psychological Association.

Hsieh, N. (2021). *Constructing bicultural identity and shame resilience in Chinese Americans* [Doctoral dissertation]. Loma Linda University).

Kim, B. K., Li, L. C., & Ng, G. F. (2005). The Asian American Values Scale--Multidimensional: Development, reliability, and validity. *Cultural Diversity and Ethnic Minority Psychology*, 11(3), 187–201. https://doi.org/10.1037/1099-9809.11.3.187

Lui, P. P., & Rollock, D. (2018). Greater than the sum of its parts: Development of a measure of collectivism among Asians. *Cultural Diversity and Ethnic Minority Psychology*, 24(2), 242–259. https://doi.org/10.1037/cdp0000163

Masuda, A., & Boone, M. S. (2011). Mental health stigma, self-concealment, and help-seeking attitudes among Asian American and European American college students with no help-seeking experience. *International Journal for the Advancement of Counseling, 33*(4), 266–279. https://doi.org/10.1007/s10447-011-9129-1

Navarrete, V., & Jenkins, S. R. (2011). Cultural homelessness, multiminority status, ethnic identity development, and self-esteem. *International Journal of Intercultural Relations, 35*(6), 791–804. https://doi.org/10.1016/j.ijintrel.2011.04.006

Shih, K. Y., Chang, T. F., & Chen, S. Y. (2019). Impacts of the model minority myth on Asian American individuals and families: Social justice and critical race feminist perspectives. *Journal of Family Theory & Review, 11*(3), 412–428. https://doi.org/10.1111/jftr.12342

Substance Abuse and Mental Health Services Administration (2023). *Asian American, Native Hawaiian, and Pacific Islander (AA and NHPI).* https://www.samhsa.gov/behavioral-health-equity/aa-nhpi.

Ting-Toomey, S. (2015). Identity negotiation theory. In J. Bennett (Ed.), *Sage encyclopedia of intercultural competence* (Vol. 1, pp. 418–422). Sage.

Tracy, J. L., Robins, R. W., & Tangney, J. P. (2007). *The self-conscious emotions: Theory and research.* The Guilford Press.

Tran, N., & Paterson, S. E. (2016). "American" as a proxy for "whiteness": Racial color-blindness in everyday life. In A. Dottolo & E. Kaschak (Eds.), *Whiteness and white privilege in psychotherapy* (1st ed., pp. 175–189). Routledge.

Tuan, M. (1998). *Forever foreigners or honorary whites? The Asian ethnic experience today.* Rutgers University Press.

Van Vliet, K. J. (2008). Shame and resilience in adulthood: A grounded theory study. *Journal of Counseling Psychology, 55*(2), 233. https://doi.org/10.1037/0022-0167.55.2.233

Wong, Y. J., Kim, B. S., Nguyen, C. P., Cheng, J. K. Y., & Saw, A. (2014). The Interpersonal shame inventory for Asian Americans: Scale development and psychometric properties. *Journal of Counseling Psychology, 61*(1), 119. https://doi.org/10.1037/a0034681.

Wong, Y., & Tsai, J. (2007). Cultural models of shame and guilt. In J. L. Tracy, R.W. Robins, & J. P. Tangney (Eds.), *The self-conscious emotions: Theory and research* (pp. 209–223). Guilford Press.

Wu, C., Qian, Y., & Wilkes, R. (2021). Anti-Asian discrimination and the Asian-white mental health gap during COVID-19. *Ethnic and Racial Studies, 44*(5), 819–835. https://doi.org/10.1080/01419870.2020.1851739

Yeh, C. J., & Hwang, M. Y. (2000). Interdependence in ethnic identity and self: Implications for theory and practice. *Journal of Counseling & Development, 78*(4), 420–429. https://doi.org/10.1002/j.1556 6676.2000.tb01925.x

# Chapter 8

# Relational Ethics at the Heart of Asian American Family Systems

*Wonyoung L. Cho*

Pain pulls for a response. When we witness someone or something in pain, something within us usually responds – in empathy, in sympathy, with remorse and guilt, or with righteous anger. These internal responses then inspire social action of some kind: efforts to comfort, aid, and/or support. We also often feel the pull to examine the context and to judge: was this pain warranted? Was it wrong? And if so, who or what is responsible? The specific details of what we judge – how we interpret and make meaning of what is expected, what is right or wrong, as well as how we should respond to such ethical dilemmas might differ across cultures, communities, and individuals. But it seems that humanity in general engages in processes of ethical considerations when making sense of and responding to pain.

There are those who believe that these benign impulses to care and to judge are innate to human nature (Rawls, 1963). This belief is also deeply rooted in many world religions. This intangible and sometimes unarticulated sense of right and wrong (in other words, a sense of justice) as well as the impulse to care is imprinted in the depths of every being. However, in this also lies a problem, especially in such a diverse and multifaceted society like the United States of America: how exactly do we determine what is right and wrong? And I do not mean the legal kind – although that too requires some serious re-examination and contemplation. How do we determine what is good and fair within the social interactions of our nuanced, relational contexts?

## Relational Ethics: What Is Good? What Is Fair?

Determining right from wrong in a relationship is never simple. It depends on who is in the relationship, what the nature of the relationship is, as well as the social, cultural, chronological, and developmental context of the individuals and the relational system. For example, what is right between a parent and a child may not be right for siblings. What was right between intimate partners last year may not be what is right between them today. And the standards guiding what might be considered relationally appropriate and ethical continue to shift quickly

DOI: 10.4324/9781003321590-12

– especially in this highly connected fast-paced technological and globalized society. There is so much noise in our lives today about how to make meaning of our relational experiences.

The diversity of perspectives and opinions on what is ethical is not new. To determine what is good, what is warranted, and what is expected then depends on our historical, sociocultural, economic, political, and spiritual contexts. The myriad of unique intersections creates a *multiplicity of good*, and it is exactly this multiplicity of good that puts us in an ethical dilemma (Gergen, 2015). For those of us who live in-between cultures like Asian Americans, even more so. The range of variables that contribute to our sense of what is fair is that much greater and ambiguous.

In Western cultural traditions, ethics are often organized around the individual (Shaw, 2011). It centers on an individual (or an individual party) and focuses on what is "authentic" or true to one's self. It often fails to consider accountability and consideration of how one's actions and choices influence and affect others. The systems that guard mental health professions and many of our theories of practice also have individuals centered in their foundations. Eastern cultural traditions as well as those who study relationships closely conceptualize ethics differently. Rather than thinking about ethics objectively at the level of the individual, ethics are often defined more relationally. What is good is determined by what is "good for us." This has a distinctively more subjective tone and has been interpreted differently over time and contexts.

However, when "us" is interpreted in a rigid and static light, this abstract and external idea of "us" becomes a dominating force that can seemingly impose standards of good and fair that may feel oppressive. In this context, what is "good for us" can be used to dictate the actions of an individual or a minority group in the name of the majority. For example, patriarchal values and heteronormative lifestyles are deemed what is "good for us" in cultures that value the continuation of the family name through procreation and bloodlines and lead to oppression and silencing of queer gender identities and sexual orientations. Thus, the relational ethics that we must pursue are not so simple and static.

### Relational Justice

Relational ethics framed through Contextual Family Therapy (Boszormenyi-Nagy & Krasner, 1986; Boszormenyi-Nagy & Spark, 1973) helps clarify what is "good for us" in a more nuanced way: "welfare and interests of every other member are taken into account by others, and individuals strive for the balance of fairness between what each member is obligated to give and entitled to receive" (Hargrave & Pfitzer, 2003, p. 10). Here, *obligated to give* and *entitled to receive* takes on a particular meaning. Because the impulse to care for others and motivation to be fair in our relationships are assumed to be in all of us (as exemplified by our innate, natural response to pain), it follows that the nature of humanity is to give and receive care from one another. It is also assumed that we have a certain innate sense of what is fair (Rawls, 1963). In other words, "good for us" should promote growth and health of the individuals in the relationship as well as the relationship itself (the "us"); and this is guided by our innate sense of relational justice.

Some Confucian theorists also offer similar interpretations – that Confucian relational ethics, often cited for organizing familial relationships into cold, strict, and patriarchal hierarchies in Sinosphere cultures, is actually "an interpersonal 'way of being with' and a 'way of social interaction'" (Wang, 2022, p. 2). Rather than diluting the complex writings and teachings of Confucius to simply legitimize patriarchal "us" as the supreme authority to determine relational ethics, his emphasis on equality of human nature, free will, and development of personal character necessitates invitation as these offer thoughtful engagement around what is good and fair in relationships. Similarly, many of the world's religious and philosophical tools used to cast relational ethics as rigid dos and shoulds are probably missing what the original sources intended, which is a careful and nuanced balancing of individuals and relationships ("us") to determine what is good and fair.

### Trustworthiness

Over the course of time, we accrue experiences that either affirm our innate sense of relational justice or disillusion it. We determine whether the world, the people in it, and those we are in relation with are *trustworthy* in the sense that they will satisfy our need for relational give and take (Hargrave & Pfitzer, 2003). In other words, we begin to engage with the world with our own set of assumptions of how trustworthy someone is in giving what we are *entitled to receive* and how much we are *obligated to give* in return. Over the course of our own lifetime, we have accrued enough experiences that we have determined how *trustworthy* our relationships are. We may not have articulated it in that particular way, but we certainly approach particular relationships with less vulnerability or with more ease than others.

Setting aside the diverse range of personalities and relational histories at the individual level, the residues of immigration and acculturation mediate our intergenerational legacies. I have witnessed many families struggle over not only the *multiplicity of good* that exists within one sociocultural context but the disconnect that comes with navigating multiple sociocultural contexts with diverse languages, cultural values, and ways of doing things. Intentions and actions get lost between translation, and what was already challenging to begin with becomes even more confusing with the plurality of a *multiplicity of good*. We are quick to interpret our elders' lack of touch as lack of emotions, their lack of words as lack of love, and indirect communication as passive aggression. Through this lens, we have come to mistake a culturally specific expression and way of giving care as lack of care. Is it possible that their giving of care has been lost in translation, and it is up to us as clinicians and following generations to develop contextually informed translation skills?

I grew up in a small city in the southwestern United States as a 1.5-generation Korean-American immigrant. As an immigrant who lived my formative years in South Korea, my country of origin, I was socialized within that culture, completed my early childhood and elementary education there, and gained mastery of my heritage language. I had the advantage of being a cultural insider that my US-born Korean-American friends did not have. As we grew older and as our urges to launch away from our families peaked, I saw acts of care get lost in translation when parents and children did not share language or culture. This is not to say I did not experience the same pressures to live out my teenage independence through the lens of assimilation. I certainly yearned for the freedom to drive at 16, to go to the movies and have sleepovers with friends, and to have a phone call with a crush without my mother listening on the other end of the line. I also yearned for expressions of care that were more congruent with the dominant culture I was socializing in – words of affirmation rather than critiques and permission to explore expression of self through dress and make-up, for example. I did not receive care in this way. However, I shared language with my parents and my parents were able to communicate to me that we must not lose connection through these fissures of bicultural pressures and of developmental stressors that our family faced. Much of my parents' care for me, despite it not being palatable to my Americanized teenage tastes, did not get lost in translation.

When we put on the individualistic lens of relational ethics, it is easy to criticize the earlier generations of immigrant families and pressure them to emulate Western ideals of parenting. We are often quick to advocate for the child struggling in the cacophony of what they are *entitled to receive* from their parents. Even when we consider relational ethics as defined in Contextual Family Therapy, it is easy to default to blaming the parents for their oppressive reign over the child's individuality because we hold the one on top of the generational hierarchy as responsible (more on this later). However, it is necessary to consider whether the parents, from their generational and cultural spaces, have in fact been *giving care* that has gotten lost in translation.

For example, my mother and I have a relationship that is stereotypically and uniquely first-born-daughter-immigrant-mother (see the *Joy Luck Club* by Amy Tan, 1989). One day, my mother pulled me aside to tell me to keep my head down when I started to post on social media about racial injustices, the Black Lives Matter movement, and critiques about the sociopolitical climate. When using the social justice framework of the US, my mother's gesture could be interpreted as colluding with the white supremacist discourse of model minority myth (Walton & Truong, 2023) and anti-blackness (Yellow Horse et al., 2021). Using a simplistic Korean sociocultural framework, my mother could be pressuring me to uphold the traditional and simplified Confucian values of patriarchy and humility. Furthermore, my mother could be demonstrating poor boundaries and overstepping into my life because she over-identifies with me and finds meaning for herself through my life and career – a story all too common for immigrant mothers who have sacrificed so much of their own individuality for her family's survival in someone else's country. All of this meaning-making can be true. And in all of these possible interpretations, my mother does not seem *trustworthy* in terms of relational ethics. None of these interpretations lend themselves to the idea that she is giving care to me as her daughter. If anything, they seem to cast her as self-serving, engaging in *destructive entitlement* (Hargrave & Anderson, 1992, as cited in Hargrave & Pfitzer, 2003) to compensate for her own unmet needs.

Before we place final judgment on my mother, there is one more plausible interpretation and we need to know a little bit about the modern history of South Korea to understand it. My mother spent her formative years in South Korea from the 1960s to 1980s. The Republic of Korea was still a nascent country following centuries of monarchy, 35 years of Japanese colonization, then the Korean War (1950–1953); and the newly liberated nation was still not quite settled into democracy. There was a military coup in 1961 and Park Chung-hee ruled for the next 17 years as the third "president" of South Korea. Another military dictator, Chun Doo-hwan, usurped the regime when Park was assassinated in 1979 and was "president" of South Korea from 1980 to 1988. During these decades of military regime, South Korea saw significant and miraculous economic growth. It also experienced significant oppression of various freedoms of the people including freedom of press and speech, discarding of individuals and groups who did not "contribute" to society. There was very little room for public critique of the regime during these decades, and many students and academics from the universities suffered and were killed in their efforts to demonstrate their opposition.

It is in this very specific sociopolitical context – which is easily lost through the fissures of immigration – my mother's gestures take on a new meaning. One of the things she said to me in Korean when she was encouraging me to keep my silence was, "the loud academics are the first to disappear." All of a sudden, her efforts to quiet me down were about her giving care to me as her daughter – about protecting me from being targeted for my ideas and ensuring my survival in an escalating sociopolitical climate. I am not obligated to submit to her requests (again, more on this later), but I am not left wanting and wounded in what I am *entitled to receive* as her child. Understanding my mother's lived history allows me to receive her care for me, even if it is not palatable to my tastes.

The reality of what transpired between me and my mother can be any and all of the above interpretations. The relationship between my mother and me as well as our individuality are embedded in the multiple meanings of our interaction. It is in this multiplicity that an ethic of care is recognized and I can understand my mother as well as our relationship complexly. This complexity enables me to see beyond the simplistic interpretation of a seemingly oppressive dynamic that needs to be "cut off," completely re-written, or overthrown.

It is impossible to know every detail of the sociopolitical, cultural, and historical contexts surrounding each family we work with as marriage and family therapists. It is very possible that some of the hurts that come from perceived lack of care is indeed warranted. However, it is critical to open up the room for such invisible stories in the Asian and Asian American families before jumping in with judgments on whether appropriate care has been given. It is crucial that we imagine the earlier generations complexly and sit with the *multiplicity of good* instead of flattening their intentions into a simple (and often inaccurate) dichotomy of *trustworthiness* from a US-based framework.

## Loyalty

In my recollection of my mother in the story above, I may be motivated by something more than just accurate event-telling. I am conscious of my *loyalty* to my mother, much like the one I hold for my family and my culture of origin. *Loyalty* in Contextual Therapy is defined as "one's sense of obligation and connection to those who have earned love and care, either by nature of their own offering of love and care or by nature of the relationship" (Schmidt et al., 2019, p. 8), and I definitely have chosen my relationship with my mother over the simpler interpretations of her actions. It is in my intentional loyalty to my mother that I seek complexity in the difficult interactions I have with her. It is my way of coping with the *multiplicity of good* and the dilemma of *split loyalty* in the sociocultural intersection of Korea, the US, Asian America, and critical epistemology.

As Asian Americans, we often experience the ethical dilemma of *split loyalty* (Boszormenyi-Nagy & Krasner, 1986 as cited in Hargrave & Pfitzer, 2003) in having to choose *loyalty* to one relationship at the cost of another. In our individual relationships with the social scripts of our culture of origin and the dominant culture of the US, we may have made various choices to cope, code-switch, assimilate, and/or resist. Perhaps this dichotomous choice of having to show *loyalty* to one culture over the other has pervaded our daily lives – in our families, in our schools and workplaces, in the grander scheme of society. And perhaps the answer to this dilemma has seemed easier in recent years as national attention and awareness of matters of diversity, equity, and inclusion has increased following the COVID-19 pandemic, the resurgence of civil rights movement, and overt rise in anti-Asian hate crimes. It is easier to see the lack of *trustworthiness* that the Asian American communities feel from the US now than it was a few years ago. However, I would like to propose that perhaps we do not have to choose at all: there is a third option.

When we sift through the *multiplicity of good* by holding multiple meaning-makings in the same space, we start to tease apart the threads that seem tangled up together. I am taking the third option to hold both and position and resist the dichotomy in my relationship with my mother: it is possible for my mother to be both caring for me and seeking to compensate for her individuality lost in the battlegrounds of immigrant life. It is possible for our elders to be both benevolent in their intentions and oppressive in their impact. It is possible for us to be *loyal* to both our families and the wider US cultural values with which we align.

In sum, intentionally framing ethics in the context of relationships articulates what is often taken for granted and forgotten: we are always living in relation to others, and others have profound effects on the way that we experience, understand, and interact with the world. Despite what popular culture and discourse would have us believe, even our self-concept of who we are is not established in a vacuum. What we consider to be an authentic self is profoundly and inevitably shaped by our audience. We also have choices in what interpretations we choose to privilege and believe (what or who to be *loyal* to); we have more than one way of interpreting and understanding others.

## Lost in Translation: Imagining Others Complexly

In order to bridge the gap between language and cultures, we need to (re)imagine our families and our elders complexly in the *multiplicity of good*. We need to imagine our own history complexly. We need to be suspicious and critically curious of the simple, whittled-down stories of our motherlands that are handed to us, and search out thickened, rich alternative stories for ourselves (White & Epston, 1990). The ability to reserve room for *multiplicity of good* grows with our experience in holding multiple, diverse, and sometimes conflicting stories in the same space. It is in this confusing and messy space that we have access to a fuller, more socioculturally appropriate and inclusive picture of relational ethics to work with families.

Sometimes, I find that we are quicker and more willing to hold *multiplicity of good* for others than for our own families and communities. In my conversations with friends and colleagues within the Asian American and Korean American communities, I have witnessed how quickly we assign totalizing descriptors to our parents, elders, and cultures of origin – perceiving them flatly as pre-modern, outdated, oppressive, cold, and restricted. However, cultures are never innately one thing; and it is never flat, rigid, or static. Culture is always evolving, flexing, and flowing. We feed it our stories, and it becomes what we say it is; the other existing elements of culture that have not been named are then obscured in time and lost in history. This is true for what we call American culture, our hybrid culture of Asia America, and our culture(s) of origin. Our stories are only as rich as what we know about our history – official and unofficial stories that shape our legacy and identities. It is up to us to inquire about the complex history of our communities.

### Organization and Hierarchy

One of the dynamics critical to relationships and relational ethics that is in dire need of a more complex definition is hierarchy. The imagery we often conjure up when we think of hierarchy is power over and submission to. Resistance is then violent revolution or a coup-d'etat in which all kinds of hierarchy are razed to the ground. In some ways, this mirrors the way the American revolution is storied in high school history classes: a detached and oppressive king from across the ocean taxed his colonies for his own profit and gain without consideration of the colonies and its people's plight, and the colonies rose up against such injustice to demand their relational rights (e.g., "no taxation without representation!"). When their demands were ignored, they had no choice but to take arms and wage war (e.g., "give me liberty or give me death!"). Then, upon their violent victory, they established a new kind of egalitarian and democratic social organization in which there would never be a king and all men are "created equal" with "certain unalienable Rights" such as "Life, Liberty, and Pursuit of Happiness" (Declaration of Independence, US 1776). In this story, all hierarchies are untrustworthy and unjust, and individual rights to live their own lives without interference trump all others (e.g., "do not tread on me").

We seem to approach a lot of relational hierarchies this way: hyperfocused on what we are *entitled to receive* and idealize a flat egalitarian dynamic in which individuals are free to be whoever they want to be. This pervades in the way we define relational and individual health, the way we define healthy boundaries, and the way we imagine *relational justice*. And in this dichotomous framework, submitting to a hierarchy and being attached to one another, to our elders, and to our community are assigned words like "co-dependent," "low differentiation," "parentification," and "poor/no boundaries." There are situations in which these words and what they mean are clinically warranted; *and* I do want to exhort us to pause and to reassess whether we have mistranslated some of the socioculturally specific relational dynamics within our communities.

Emotional or relational violent coup d'etat in our families against our elders is not the single correct answer to tangled hierarchies, burdened by the intergenerational traumas from our motherlands and the immigration journey. Furthermore, a complete rejection of hierarchy in pursuit of some utopian, egalitarian anarchy is not the only alternative. We need to reimagine relational hierarchies. I believe there are benevolent hierarchies – ones responsive to checks and balances, where those in the upper tiers are accountable, open, and responsive to feedback; and where those on the lower tiers are equally responsible and active in keeping the giving and taking of care in fair balance.

## In the Context of Time: Participation and Negotiation in Relational Hierarchy

Benevolent hierarchy is easier to imagine in particular phases of a family's development. When a two-generation family has children who are early in their physical, emotional, and cognitive development and under the care of adults who are physically, emotionally, and cognitively more advanced, it is plain to see how hierarchy can be benevolent, helpful, and necessary. Contextual Family Therapy names these as *vertical relationships* (Hargrave & Pfitzer, 2003) and defines the uneven, one-sided giving as "fair" and "balanced." Here, the giving and taking of care is unidirectional and generally accepted as the norm. It would be absurd and unfair to hold a five-year-old responsible to contribute financially to the family. The ways in which the five-year-old would be expected to participate in the family should be developmentally appropriate and ultimately for the child's good rather than the good of their caretaker. This is because what is *good for us* in this *vertical relationship* should also be good for the child, meet their developmental needs, and further encourage acquisition of skills and knowledge.

Relational justice starts to become murky as the relational variables start to vary. When considering adult children, what may be considered fair in a *vertical relationship* may not be so objectively clear because giving of care becomes bidirectional. Furthermore, the elders are *entitled to receive* care throughout their lives. In my *loyalty* to our community, I might argue that giving of care through seeing, honoring, and respecting our elders as the following generation is even more crucial as our elders are disconnected from their own stories, families, and communities of origin and then often erased, disrespected, and cast aside by the anti-Asian discourse in the US. What our elders are *entitled to receive* as humans is often not given, and their innate need to be cared for is not met.

I think as children of immigrants, we somehow sense this deficit of care our elders receive early on. In immigrant families where the children quickly become more knowledgeable about sociocultural norms and language of the new country, the child(ren) give care to their elders and families earlier as cultural and linguistic brokers because of practicality. We are needed to translate at medical appointments, banks, school engagements, and translate the mail for our parents whose cultural capital in the US is limited. Thus, this is how our experiences are storied through individual-oriented ethics: our immigrant parents have cast us with more responsibilities than developmentally and socially appropriate, infringing on our rights as children to enjoy our individual and self-focused development. Perhaps this version of the story is true, they have failed us in that particular way. And perhaps, through relational ethics, that is not the only way to understand what has happened between us and our elders.

The social systems such as the educational, financial, and medical institutions in the US did not make an alternative resource available for our elders. These systems may have participated in encouraging the children to fill in the gap.

Furthermore, it is not uncommon for families and societies to expect its younger members to contribute; other societies and cultures recognize the younger members' *obligation to give* also. For example, it is not uncommon for children to have considerable responsibility in doing farming chores in rural communities, or for older siblings to care for their younger ones, or for the youth to yield their comfortable chairs in public transportation to the elders. When we decenter the individualistic or Western ways of thinking about *vertical relationships*, completely unidirectional giving of care is no longer the norm.

Expectations in *vertical relationships* should be filtered through the *multiplicity of good* and understood over time. Rather than holding the elders as static givers of care and solely responsible, both parties (us and our elders) should be both accountable to the tending of the relationship – and this ratio of giving and taking of care is negotiated and gradually adjusted over time. If what is good is determined by what is good for us, it should follow that "us" is dependent on the individuals who make up the "us." Thus, what is good for us across time should adjust and change according to the younger who begin to age and start developing their own individuality, the elder whose needs and abilities also change as they age, and the relationship that flux accordingly. Ideally, as the elder(s) give room in the relationship for the younger to develop their individuality, the younger also start growing into their own *obligation to give* back to the relationship in the forms of respectful deference and attentive audience.

Here, I want to highlight the difference between respectful deference and undifferentiated submission in the context of relational ethics. Respectful deference in relational accountability extends the benefit of doubt. We hold the possibility that their intentions may be good and based on their *obligation to give* care and that it has been lost in translation. We are *obligated to give* room (and time) for their intentions to make their way over to us across fissures of immigration and through the sociocultural, linguistic, and generational gaps. And when we finally hear and see it, we are *obligated to give* communication that we have received their good intentions.

For example, I mentioned I am not obligated to submit to my mother's requests of keeping silent in my earlier story about the exchange between my mother and me. My *obligation to give* to my mother in our relationship is satisfied when I receive her care which I am *entitled to receive* and communicate to her that I have received it. Then, in determining what is *good for us*, our relationship has to also make room for what is good for me individually – which at that point in my life as a young adult was to make my own choices by considering my current sociocultural and political contexts, my relationship to the wider US culture, my personal and professional obligations to others in my life, as well as her advice in her care for me. My resistance to completely submitting to my mother's request is "good for us" because it is good for my individuality. And ultimately, I know based on the *trustworthiness* of our relationship and the mutual *loyalty* we have to one another that my mother also wants what is good for my individuality (even if it is not palatable to her tastes). I have contributed to the health and ethics of our relationship by resisting the pull for one-sided power and control.

That is not to say intentions do not excuse impact. The harmful impact of words, behaviors, and/or actions needs accountability, no matter how good and benign the intention was. There is always a cost to painful impact, and that cost needs to be accounted for somehow. However, I want to resist the totalizing idea that intentions completely do not matter. Just as intentions do not excuse impact, impact does not always override intentions.

## Relational Ethics of Power and Its Management

Ethics guide the use and management of power, and elements of power are easier to identify when considering systemic structures on the meso- and macro-levels of society. Powers that are assigned to a position by social agreement are seemingly more static and relatively easier to identify. These are the kinds of structural power that come with particular positions. For example, there is capital and thus power that comes with being a legal adult or being documented; power that comes with being of higher social class with access to resources and money; there are social powers and default deference given to male-bodied folx in patriarchy, heterosexual folx in heteronormativity, and white-presenting folx in white supremacy. These kinds of power are held regardless of merit and granted by society through an implicit social agreement and assumption. The current social justice narratives focus on these structural powers, rightfully so, and ask individuals given these kinds of power to be more aware and accountable to the others who have less of it (Combs, 2019; Watson, 2019; Watson et al., 2020).

There is another element of power that also needs to be considered when examining relationships at the micro-level. There is a softer and less visible kind of power that is more fluid unlike structural power discussed above. When two or more individuals from unique facets of identities with various structural powers connect in a relationship, a particular dimension of power develops within the relationship between the individuals. This kind of power flexes moment to moment as the various dimensions of individuals' identities move to the fore depending on the context, the nature of, and the moment in the relationship. Relational ethics then take on and guide the precarious balancing act of this relational power, which needs to be tended to from all ends of the relationship. Relational power also waxes and wanes moment to moment, and it is important for MFTs to track its movement and patterns to understand the nuanced power dynamic of the relationship(s) (ChenFeng et al., 2017; Knudson et al., 2015).

The tricky variable is that often, relational power is invisible to those who do not work to see it. Moreover, those who hold power often do not know they do until it is taken. In other words, power is best recognized by those who it affects and through its impact rather than those who wield it. And because those who hold power often do not know they have it, passing on to or sharing with another can often become a struggle. This seems especially true when we correlate organizational hierarchy to age as well as power, as though hierarchy is organized as a pyramid with elders and power naturally concentrated up at the top. However, this static and structural source of relational power is a myth – the power at the top comes from the implicit social agreement and deference. Power in hierarchies, relational, structural, or otherwise, often sits in the middle – with those who are young enough and old enough to move into and hold societal and structural capital. Power at the top of the pyramid is only possible when those at the middle knowingly or unknowingly agree to defer to those at the top.

Power in relationships is influenced by the context, specifically the context of structural power that individuals in the family are given by society. Structural power often resides in a societal position (e.g., voting power, earning capital, being documented, and so on). Thus, it is usually the generation that is in their middle adulthood who holds positions in society that gives them societal and social capital. It follows then that those who are in this season of life hold most of the relational power in the family. Those who age into late adulthood lose the kind of structural power as our society encourages them into retirement and off of society's stage. As they lose relevance to the sociocultural context around them, they may start to feel the loss of power that they forgot they had. There naturally may be grief and resistance as the power gets passed on. If they engage in the relational ethics and remember their *obligation to give* to those who come up after them, they may more gracefully acquiesce in the transition of structural power. If it is not freely given, then the younger who are moving into their adulthood will be moved to fight for what they are *entitled to receive.*

Similarly, those who come up into adulthood are *obligated to give* care to those who are grieving as they phase out of power. Rather than casting the older generation aside and forcefully retiring them out of relevance, we can give care by listening to their stories and respecting their legacies. While we are not obligated to acquiesce in all of their advice, demands, and/or requests, it is important to communicate to them that we have received their care, hear their stories, and honor their experiences. Furthermore, as increased power comes with increased *obligations to give*, those who moved into power need to keep their eyes on the *obligation to give* to those who come after and work to not forget to relinquish this power when their time comes. Thus, rather than power and time (age) being a correlated rise with no end (see Figure 8.1), power seems to rise, peak, and then fall more like a bell curve (see Figure 8.2). As such, rather than power having to be won and usurped, it should be more or less naturally passed at points in which the lines of different generations meet in Figure 8.2. This would capture the balance of both *entitlement to receive* and *obligation to give*, as well as the changing roles in the obligations that come with fluxing structural and societal power.

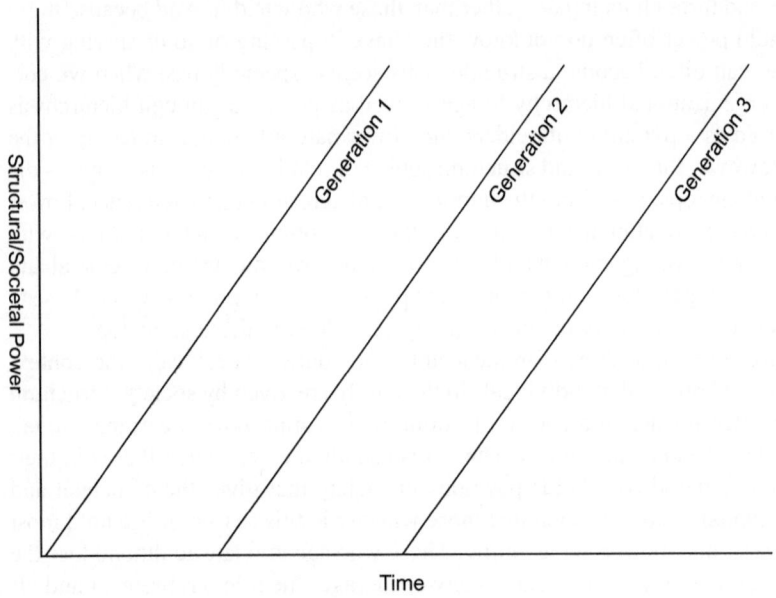

*Figure 8.1* Power as linear growth

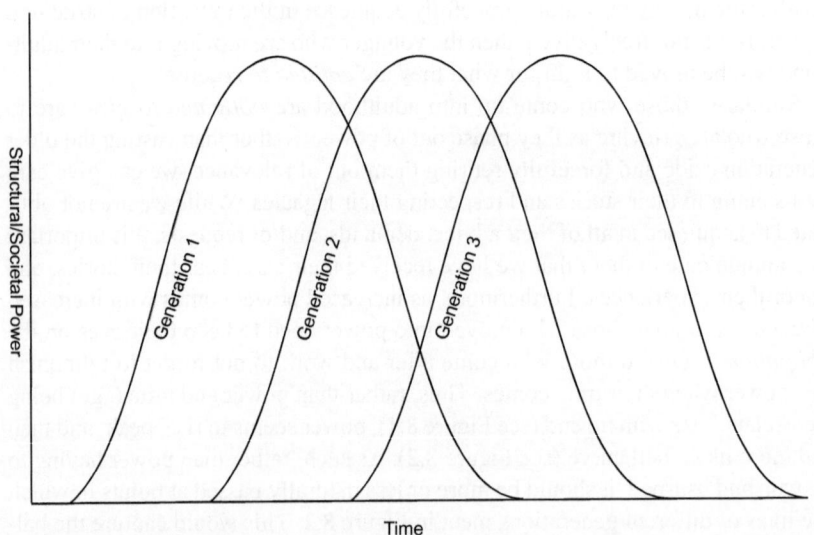

*Figure 8.2* Power as a bell curve

When what is good for us is considered by all generations involved, the previous generation should consider scaffolding, sharing, and ultimately passing the torch and the following generation should consider ways to continue honoring and remembering the legacy of the generations before. There is grief in the passing, the celebration in remembering, and hope in what is to come. This is different from throwing out the hierarchy completely. Rather, this involves taking complete accountability for the power that waxes and wanes between relationships and through various developmental phases of the family system.

The dynamics of relational power impacted by immigration has additional layers to consider. Often, the children in immigrant families – especially those who have been identified as the caretaker – take up relational power earlier than their counterparts in other families. This is because they have more societal and structural power than the adults in the family, who are disempowered due to lack of language, sociocultural knowledge, and access to social capital such as education and resources. The balance of *obligation to give* and *entitlement to receive* care has been compromised.

Families respond differently to such disruption. The parents may become more aggressive and rigid in their hold for relational power over their children to make up for this loss of power and influence, perhaps for their own sense of self or perhaps in their own efforts to *give care* to their children. In this survival stance, their bid and hold on relational power may have started out seeking what is "good for us," but have not been adjusted and negotiated with the changing needs and developmental stages of the family.

There may be regret – for the adults who did not have the resources and societal power to *give care* the way they may have wished, and for the children who did not receive what they are *entitled to receive* in the battlegrounds of immigrant life. It is important to note that this is not due to lack of desire or motivation; the relational ethics framework helps put this impossible situation in the context of the macro-, meso-, and micro-levels of power and relational dynamics rather than placing the blame on an individual (namely, the adult who failed to provide what the children are *entitled to receive*). Furthermore, holding *multiplicity of good*, we can look for other ways that care has been given and look for ways to balance the ledger of care.

### Abuse of Relational Power

There are situations, however, in which good intentions cannot account for damaging impact. When power is repeatedly misused and for prolonged periods of time, it can leave a lasting impact on the relationship and the individuals involved in that relationship, creating a kind of *debt* that cannot be absolved. Not all relationships can be restored through contextualizing care with a new found understanding of what has been done and what has come to be. In some cases, it is not care lost in translation. It actually is a lack of care, and the involved individuals or parties are not interested, available, or able to re-negotiate, salvage, and restore the relationship. In these cases, it is understandable and necessary to focus on moving forward without carrying the burden of such hurtful, abusive relationships. It may even be more beneficial to the next generation and ethical for others in the present that such draining relationships are "sealed off." This would help salvage other relationships from the damaging effects of *destructive entitlement* that such relational debt can trigger.

## Clinical Example

Sunny (age 25) is a Korean-American young cis-female professional who began therapy following the recent death of Sunny's paternal grandfather, an important patriarch in the family. He died after a long battle with cancer, and Sunny and her family attended the three-day funeral in South Korea. She reports difficulty concentrating at work and randomly bursting into tears. Furthermore, she reports that stressors at home have increased: her father has been feeling "heavy" emotionally and his usually conservative restrictions on her life have heightened, including the strictness of her curfew, especially after her grandfather's death.

Sunny has been living with her parents and her younger brother after graduating college, since her parents requested that she move back in with them. She has been increasingly supporting her family by tending to housework while continuing at her own corporate job so that her parents could focus on their business. When asked about her choices to live with her parents, she shrugged and reported that this is what is culturally expected and it is helpful for her financially. When asked about the dynamics at home, Sunny reports that she does a lot of the household chores as her parents are often tired from working manual labor, and her brother is not really helpful around the house. She described being parentified at a young age, translating for her parents, and taking care of her younger brother.

The therapist was careful not to problematize Sunny's parentified experience and explored her relationship with her parents and her grandfather whom she is currently mourning by creating a genogram with Sunny. Through the genogram, Sunny was able to articulate that she perceived her grandfather as a parental figure, someone from whom she could count on to receive care that she was *entitled to receive*. "I can't expect to be cared for by my parents the way I am cared for by my grandfather," she said in one session, "My parents are starting to feel like my children, like I have to look out for and take care of them. Maybe it felt like that way before but I just didn't think about it like this."

The therapist explored the context of immigrant life and experience, the disempowerment one experiences as they try to navigate a society that was not made for them, and how this may compromise Sunny's parents' ability to provide care for their children. Sunny then compared this to her grandfather, who she always saw in the context of her motherland, where he was established and well connected – and ultimately able to provide the kind of care that a parent or an elder would provide to their children to Sunny. As the therapist worked with Sunny to exonerate her parents from the lack of care that Sunny experienced and continues to experience, the therapist also grieved with Sunny for not having the kind of carefree childhood that she desired. In this context, Sunny's grief due to her grandfather's passing was more palpable – as though she herself lost a parent.

Next, the therapist and Sunny worked through Sunny's frustration at the increased monitoring and restrictions in her life, posed by her father at the wake of her grandfather's passing. "This kind of care feels a little late," Sunny observed one session, "I'm not a child anymore. I've never really been." As the therapist continued to hold space for Sunny's anger and frustration, the therapist expressed curiosity around her father's increased surveillance and emotional "heaviness." Sunny described her father often sitting with a faraway look – describing some kind of dissociation and general flat affect. The therapist then revisited the genogram and asked questions about the relationship between her father and her grandfather.

Threading together memories that Sunny had of her father and grandfather, as well as some "homework" for Sunny to ask her father about her grandfather, a new story started to emerge. Though her grandfather was warm, supportive, and dependable for Sunny, she also remembered moments when she would be scared of her grandfather – she described that when he had a stern look, she felt her stomach tie up in an icy knot. The stories she heard from her father highlighted this other side of her grandfather that Sunny had forgotten. Sunny started to suspect that her father was physically and emotionally abused by her grandfather. She had reported to the therapist that her father had asked her privately, "was he [her grandfather] really that wonderful of a person?" Sunny recalled this moment with newfound suspicion that her grandfather was not as warm and supportive a parent to her father as he was to her.

The therapist facilitated space for Sunny to consider the *debt* of care that her grandfather had incurred for her father, and how this may affect his ability or resources to then extend the kind of care and support that Sunny wanted from her father. Perhaps Sunny's father was attempting to care for Sunny after all, and the restrictions on her life were his own way to care for her by "keeping her safe" in the stern and conservative style he had learned from his own father. This softened Sunny to her father's care and provided space for her to consider her response rather than being reactive in anger and frustration.

Next, the therapist explored Sunny's wants and needs, how she could communicate to her father that she received his care *and* redirect his misdirected care. How could she negotiate for herself and with her father to attend to her own wellness as what is good for her is also good for him and good for their relationship ("good for us")? How could she find ways to honor her father's experience and efforts and tend to her own needs? How could she effectively negotiate the social and relational power for herself as she continues to her adulthood, and as her parents start phasing out of theirs? This process continues to require creativity and patience, but Sunny continues to find new ways to honor the hierarchy in her life without becoming disempowered and oppressed by it.

## Reflection Questions

### Questions for the Therapist

- What are some automatic assumptions you make when you consider elders from your community? What are some automatic reactions, images, and thoughts you have when thinking about your parents and elders in your community? And what informs these notions?
- Are you operating out of debt or deficit of care? Have you received the kind of care that you wanted or needed? What kind of care would you have wanted instead?
- Is there a possibility that the care your parents or caretakers provided was lost in translation? What are some sociopolitical, historical, and/or cultural contexts that would shed new light on their efforts to care for you?

### Questions for Therapy

- How does the personal reflections from above inform your blindspots as a therapist working with clients from your own community? or other immigrant and migrant communities?
- As history and personal stories shift depending on who is telling the story, how could you get exposed to complex and multifaceted stories and histories of the communities you are working with? How can you get exposed to diverse authors and storytellers to expand your ability to hold multiple and sometimes conflicting stories in the same room?

## References

Boszormenyi-Nagy, I., & Krasner, B. R. (1986). *Between give and take: A clinical guide to contextual therapy*. Brunner/Mazel.

Boszormenyi-Nagy, I., & Spark, G. M. (1973). *Invisible loyalties: Reciprocity in intergenerational family therapy*. Harper & Row (reprinted by Brunner/Mazel, 1984).

ChenFeng, J., Kim, L., Wu, Y., & Knudson-Martin, C. (2017). Addressing culture, gender, and power with Asian American couples: Application of socio-emotional relationship therapy. *Family Process, 56*(3), 558–573. https://doi.org/10.1111/famp.12251

Combs, G. (2019). White privilege: What's a family therapist to do? *Journal of Marital and Family Therapy, 45*(1), 61–75. https://doi.org/10.1111/jmft.12330

Gergen, K. J. (2015). Relational ethics in therapeutic practice. *Australian & New Zealand Journal of Family Therapy, 36*(4), 409–418. https://doi.org/10.1002/anzf.1123

Hargrave, T. D. & Pfitzer, F. (2003). *The new contextual therapy: Guiding the power of give and take.* Routledge.

Knudson, C., Huenergardt, D., Lafontant, K., Bishop, L., Schaepper, J., & Wells, M. (2015). Competencies for addressing gender and power in couple therapy: A Socio emotional approach. *Journal of Marital & Family Therapy, 41*(2) 205–220. https://doi.org/10.1111/jmft.12068

Rawls, J. (1963). The sense of justice. *The Philosophical Review, 72*(3), 281–305. https://doi.org/10.2307/2183165

Schmidt Hulst, A. E. & Sibley, D. S. (2019). *Contextual therapy for family health: Clinical applications.* Routledge.

Shaw, E. (2011). Relational ethics and moral imagination in contemporary systemic practice. *Australian & New Zealand Journal of Family Therapy, 32*(1), 1–14. https://doi.org/10.1375/anft.32.1.1

Walton, J. & Truong, M. (2023) A review of the model minority myth: understanding the social, educational and health impacts. *Ethnic and Racial Studies, 46*(3), 391–419. https://doi.org/10.1080/01419870.2022.2121170

Wang, Z. (2022). The multiple dimensions of Confucian relational ethics and the "Way of Being With." *Religions, 13*(10), 922. https://doi.org/10.3390/rel13100922

Watson, M. F. (2019). Social justice and race in the United States: Key issues and challenges for couple and family therapy. *Family Process, 58*(1), 23–33. https://doi.org/10.1111/famp.12427

Watson, M. F., Turner, W. L., & Hines, P. M. (2020). Black Lives Matter: We are in the same storm but we are not in the same boat. *Family Process, 59*(4), 1362–1373. https://doi.org/10.1111/famp.12613

White, M., & Epston, D. (1990). *Narrative means to therapeutic ends.* W.W. Norton & Company.

Yellow Horse, A. J., Kuo, K., Seaton, E. K., & Vargas, E. D. (2021). Asian Americans' indifference to Black Lives Matter: The role of nativity, belonging and acknowledgment of anti-Black racism. *Social Sciences, 10*(5), 168. https://doi.org/10.1111/famp.12613

Chapter 9

# The Next Generation
## Evolution of Asian American Identity in the Face of the U.S.'s Racial Justice Movement

*Amy Tuttle*

*In talking to people, in listening to the way they see themselves, how they grew up, their views, I was struck by the power of the larger society in influencing Asian American thinking and behavior. Asian attitudes – how Asians see themselves, how they feel they are seen by the larger society, how they want to be seen – are in large part a product of environment.*

*(Lee, 1992, p. viii)*

Asian Americans share rich traditions, values, histories, and migration legacies, and each individual, family, and community is unique with distinct qualities and identities. Asian American identity is diverse, and it is an overlooked, under-researched relational and sociopolitical process that is experienced in unique and complex ways. First-generation Asian American immigrants to the United States have very different experiences, stories, and histories from that of their third-generation grandchildren, and starkly different experiences from that of their fourth-generation great-grandchildren. To further complicate the process of Asian American identity development in second-, third-, and fourth-generations, sociopolitical issues, racial justice movements, and varied ways of retelling and recalling history impact relationships and communication in Asian American families. The evolution of Asian American identity through the third- and fourth-generations is rich and diverse, yet, it has become complex and fluid. The effects of an evolving, ever-changing Asian American identity for third- and fourth-generations have implications for relationships, communities, and visibility of Asian Americans in the United States.

## Theoretical/Conceptual Background

The evolution of Asian American identity in the third- and fourth-generations may be approached from a variety of lenses and frameworks. In this chapter, Asian American identity will be discussed and considered from a relational, sociocultural, and social constructionist framework. From this framework and perspective, Asian American identity is experienced and negotiated in relationships and

DOI: 10.4324/9781003321590-13

is impacted by history, politics, culture, family relationships, and communication. Identity is viewed and experienced as a fluid process that is impacted by others. Relational and family stories are essential to understanding one's experience of identity, and interactions between generations are explored in the context of Asian American identity in third and fourth-generations. Asian American identity is a complex relational, sociocultural process.

## Asian Americans in the United States

*Prior to the social and political upheavals of the 1960s, there was no "Asian America"—at least not as we know it today. While Americans of Asian descent had joined forces on the picket line and plantation field throughout history, their identities and struggles were mostly defined along distinct ethnic lines. But amidst the tumult of the civil rights movement, young people united their communities to forge a new identity based on their collective experiences as Asian Americans ... Yuji Ichioka, who taught the first Asian American studies class at UCLA, is credited with coining the term "Asian American" in 1968.*

*(Wallace, 2017, para. 1)*

The term Asian American includes a myriad of different ethnic and cultural groups with most people identifying their origins from East and Southeast Asia and the Indian subcontinent. Asian Americans identify as Chinese, Taiwanese, Indian, Filipino, Vietnamese, Korean, Japanese, Pakistani, Thai, Cambodian, Hmong, Laotian, Bangladeshi, Nepalese, Burmese, Indonesian, Sri Lankan, Malaysian, Mongolian, Bhutanese, and Okinawan, and they trace their roots and ancestry to more than 20 countries (Pew Research, 2021). Eighty-five percent of Asian Americans identify their origin as Chinese, Indian, Filipino, Vietnamese, Korean, and Japanese, and nearly half of all Asian Americans reside in the western United States (Pew Research, 2021). Asian populations in the United States almost doubled between 2000 and 2019, and these numbers are expected to increase.

In considering the increase of Asian Americans in the United States, psychologists, sociologists, and other researchers have examined Asian American racial and cultural identity development. Thus, there are various ways to conceptualize and approach Asian American identity development and the stages, steps, and phases one experiences based on their generation and acculturation (e.g., Kim, 1981, 2001; Sue & Sue, 1990). Kim's (1981, 2001) Asian American Identity Development Model examines age and development and includes several stages: ethnic awareness, white identification, social political consciousness, reconnection to culture and heritage, and incorporation of identity. Sue and Sue (1990) introduce stages and attitudes in their Minority Identity Development (MID) model highlighting conformity, dissonance, resistance and immersion, introspection, articulation, and awareness. In 2021, Yoo, Gabriel, Atkin, Matriano, and Akhter introduce the Asian American Racial Identity Ideological Values (AARIIV) drawing on Asian Critical Race Theory and Asian American histories of oppression and resilience. Other research has examined internal and external ethnic identity. Kwan and Sodowsky (1997) made a distinction between the two in which one's internal sense of ethnic identity was related to cognitions, morals, and affect, and external ethnic identity associated with behaviors and participation in traditions. Asian American identity research continues to evolve and more intentionally integrate the complexity of Asian American identity.

Research and literature on Asian American identity development may be enriched by researchers' contextual considerations as they relate to identity based on generation. Attias-Donfut (2015, 2016), a sociologist from France, researches these ideas and the work of Marcus Lee Hansen. In the early and mid-1900s, Hansen introduced the idea of "third-generation interest" or "third-generation return," suggesting that the second-generation assimilates to the cultural norms and expectation of the dominant culture, and the third-generation expresses an interest in a return to their grandparents' generation (e.g., Attias-Donfut, 2015, 2016). Hansen's proposal has been debated and others (e.g., Newton et al., 1988) have supported and proposed the idea that there is a gradual decrease of identification with culture based on generation. Thus, approaching Asian American identity with attention to generation and context and identity occurring in stages, phases, or prescribed models may be problematic. Perhaps Asian American identity in the third- and fourth-generations has evolved and become more fluid. Perhaps Asian American ethnic identity is "less a function of time and generational position" and more a function of one's "position in complex societies" (Newton et al., 1988, p. 305). The evolution of Asian American identity suggests a more salient role of power, privilege, and context in the process and experience of Asian American identity.

When considering Asian American identity, it is important to consider identity within the context of racial, social, and political tensions that impact individuals, communities, and relationships. In these ever-changing sociopolitical, cultural, relational landscapes, third- and fourth-generation Asian American identified people have been faced with challenge, tension, and complexity in responding to the questions of identity: *Who am I? Where do I belong?* Thus, the question and questions of identity for third- and fourth-generation Asian Americans can be a complex web of power, sociocultural and political processes, and privilege. Who *gets* to name one's identity? How do *you* see me? What do *you* see when you look at me? All of these questions have implications and impact one's view of self and one's place in our communities, in society, and in the United States.

Though there have been invaluable contributions to better understanding Asian American identity, Asian American racial identity development is a fluid process that is directly influenced by sociopolitical, relational, and historical factors and relationships. Therefore, applying identity to a set of stages and phases becomes problematic. Racial and ethnic identity construction in Asian Americans is also informed by self *and* other, and the identity construction process may be markedly different in each generation. Is identity construction different because of an increasing distance from family migration legacies? Is this difference related to the increased representation and upward mobility of Asian Americans in U.S. American society? Is increased Asian American representation and upward mobility a reality or is it a socially constructed myth? Are there truly marked differences in identity by generation? Are there similarities in racial identity construction between generations? Who *gets* to decide?

The increased distance from family migration stories may contribute to different racial identity construction processes. However, how can we understand this distance? Who is responsible for the distance? *What* is responsible for the distance? Racism, race-related fear, shame, and trauma are powerful and collude with the dominant culture to create systems of oppression and silence, thus overpowering communication and relationships. Family race and migration stories may not be discussed in families (e.g., Young et al., 2021); however, Asian American experiences and histories are embedded in systemic oppression, institutional oppressive systems, and racist political and social policies and practices that are often excluded from the retelling of U.S. history. Which histories are privileged and what impact does this have on Asian American identity?

Many believe there is increased representation of Asian Americans in the United States (e.g., Lee & Sheng, 2023); however, the ideas that Asian Americans are on the rise, they are "honorary Whites," and they are "model minorities" may be viewed as destructive myths. Lee (1992) writes that "depending on domestic economic and global political conditions, some Asian Americans are accepted as full and equal citizens in the United States while others find themselves marginalized as dangerous outsiders" (p. 374). Not all Asian Americans are on the rise, and not all ethnic groups are equally represented in leadership and in social and political realms (e.g., Goon et al., 2022), and highlighting the success of some "obscures the significant proportion of Asian Americans who still struggle to survive, live in poverty, are unemployed or underemployed, and have low rates of education" (Lee, 1992, p. 376). The rise of Asian Americans may be accurate for some; however, Asian Americans are much more diverse and are perhaps more accurately referred to as a "community of contrasts" (Lee, 1992).

### Connection to Family Migration Legacies

*Suye, was the first picture bride in Uozu, Japan to immigrate to the United States. Toajiro Ogawa, worked on the railroads in Mexico. The two married and moved to Oregon where they had six children: Kiyo, Heidi, June,*

*Masao, Lois, and Mary. When Heidi was in grade school, her teacher changed the spelling of her name to a "more phonetic spelling," H-E-I-D-E, thus, allowing the teacher to pronounce her name with ease. In 1942, the Ogawa family was forced to leave their home and successful strawberry farm, and they traveled by train to a Japanese American internment camp in Tule Lake, California where they were incarcerated for four years.*

*(Author)*

As early as the mid-1800s Asian Americans immigrated to the United States as laborers, and they made a significant impact on the development of the United States. Immigrants from China, Korea, Japan, the Philippines, and other Asian countries worked as miners, railroad builders, agricultural workers, factory workers, and fishermen (Asian Society, 2023). These early migrations to the United States led to anti-Asian legislation, discrimination, and oppressive racist policies and practices, thus, impacting Asian American identity, family stories, and legacies. Asian American stories of migration were shared with younger generations; however, as the first-generation assimilated to the dominant culture and navigated an anti-Asian environment, much of the language and these early stories of struggle, triumph, and resilience grew silent (e.g., Nagata, 1991). The stories that endured were stories of how to "fit in," how to assimilate, adjust, and accommodate to the dominant culture.

Some first-generation Asian Americans left their countries of origin in search of a "better life" and to live the American dream, and their children were born as Asian *and* American (e.g., Lee, 1992). Many in the second-generation may recall the family migration stories; however, they were now experiencing life in American culture and the oppressive, racist practices that followed. Many second-generation Asian Americans spoke their native language, and also learned English, and they became more American than their foreign-born parents. The migration legacies and precious memories and stories that brought their parents to the United States became less important; they became more hidden and silent.

In some Asian American families, migration stories are mixed with issues of racism and injustice. For instance, first-, second-, and some third-generation Japanese Americans were incarcerated from 1942 to 1946, and when they were released, silence surrounded their experiences of racism and injustice. Racism, injustice, and discrimination dominated the family's identity; thus, being Asian American and being Japanese and Japanese American was filled with shame, confusion, and distress. For example, some third-generation Japanese American children learned to stay silent and avoid topics surrounding the Japanese American incarceration during World War II. In some families, when topics related to the "camp" emerged, first-generation parents began speaking in Japanese, thus interrupting communication and connection with their children and others. Without much effort or intention, the third- and fourth-generations learned that issues of race and discrimination were not topics to engage. However, with racial justice movements in the 1960s and 1970s and the more recent racial uprising in 2020, third- and fourth-generation Asian Americans reclaimed space and voice in identity, race-related discrimination, justice, equity, and activism.

Asian American families carry different immigration and migration stories, and each family has different historical backgrounds, legacies, and experiences of racism and oppression. These stories may and may not be shared and discussed; however, when they are shared, how the stories are re-told changes and evolves with time. Silence and re-tellings are also influenced by racism and racial justice movements.

## Racism and Racial Justice Movements

Asian Americans and social activism have been sparsely published (e.g., Lui et al., 2008; Maeda, 2012; Wei, 1993). However, Asian Americans have been involved in activism and social change as early as the 1960s and 1970s. Namely, Asian American college students along the west coast demanded ethnic and Asian American studies' programs and inclusion of Asian American instructors and administration at San Francisco State College, University of California Berkeley, University of Hawai'i Manoa, and Seattle Central Community College (Maeda, 2012). At around the same time and throughout the United States, Asian American activism sought to improve conditions and access to resources in Seattle, Los Angeles, New York, and Philadelphia (Maeda, 2012). Many of these Asian American activist movements brought together other minorities and people of color, joining their efforts and forces against institutionalized racist practices, policies, and norms. Asian American activists "sought to find similarities between different ethnic, racial, and national groups around which to organize" (Maeda, 2012, p. 136).

In addition to the collaboration with other minority groups, in the 1960s, the Asian American Political Alliance at the University of California, Berkeley, brought Asian Americans together, regardless of their ethnic differences (Maeda, 2012). Asian American identity was defined by Asian American unity, interracial solidarity and transnational critical consciousness, and the shared experiences of discrimination and oppression of all Asians (Maeda, 2009, 2012). Interracial solidarity valued Asian Americans within the context of other racial groups, as well as the connections with African Americans and Blacks, solidarity and shared oppression, and a rejection of the model minority myth (Maeda, 2012). Transnational critical consciousness highlighted the shared experiences of racism and oppression between Asian and Asian Americans as a result of white supremacy and the recognition of the oppression felt by Asians globally (Lee, 1992; Maeda, 2009).

These early Asian American activists and racial justice movements paved the way for Asian Americans and people of color to unite in response to the increase of anti-Asian hate reports in 2020. Between March 2020 and March 2022, Stop

AAPI Hate received 11,500 hate incidents, and 67% of these incidents included harassment, and 17% included physical violence. Anti-Asian hate crimes increased in the early stages of the COVID-19 pandemic (Han et al., 2023).

In response to the alarming escalation in xenophobia and bigotry resulting from the COVID-19 pandemic, AAPI Equity Alliance (AAPI Equity), Chinese for Affirmative Action (CAA), and the Asian American Studies Department of San Francisco State University launched the Stop AAPI Hate coalition on March 19, 2020. The coalition tracks and responds to incidents of hate, violence, harassment, discrimination, shunning, and child bullying against Asians, Asian Americans, and Pacific Islanders (https://stopaapihate.org/about/). This surge in violence and hate incidents led to fear and increasing mental health issues and an increase in racism and discrimination toward Asian Americans (e.g., Lee & Rose, 2022).

Anti-Asian hate in 2020 emerged in the shadows of a long history of racism, oppression, and discrimination toward Asians and Asian Americans, and for many families the explicit reemergence of anti-Asian sentiments was devastating, retraumatizing, and dehumanizing. However, with changes in Asian American identity, the voices of the older generations of Asian American activists, and a new generation of Asian American voices, awareness, and openings for healing conversations and sharing stories of resilience, strength, and perseverance were possible for families and in society. Thus, communication between generations during the COVID-19 pandemic and discussions on race and racism were becoming more connected and unified (e.g., Lee & Rose, 2022). However, these conversations are not without consequence, and some families continue to avoid conversations regarding race and racism (e.g., Young et al., 2021).

The post-2020 racial uprising and racial justice movement created openings for conversations about race and racism in Asian American families. This opening for explicit conversation is healing for some families. Families are able to recall the strengths of their ancestors and first-generation immigrants to the United States. They are able to retell the stories of resilience and strength. However, these stories may also include painful recollections of racism and race-related trauma, as well as experiences of institutionalized and internalized racism that may be harder to recognize and name. Internalized forms of racism reignited painful internal, silent struggles for some Asian Americans. For instance, painful stories of Asian Americans altering their appearance to look "more American" and the medical doctors colluding with dominant views on beauty encouraging eyelid surgeries resurfaced, and the trauma of racism reexperienced in new ways and in younger generations of Asian Americans.

Historical and more recent racial uprisings and racial justice movements are beneficial in inviting younger generations to join activist movements, making anti-Asian American hate and oppression visible, and creating opportunities to confront and combat the sociopolitical forces that impede Asian American identities to flourish in the United States. It would, however, be remiss to not make visible the cost and the toll that these efforts and these conversations take on Asian Americans. Explicit and healing conversations on combating Anti-Asian hate and celebrating acts of racial activism are rich and meaningful and can also expose painful memories and ongoing internal Asian American ethnic identity struggles.

## Intergenerational Relationships and Communication

*As a child, my grandmother and grandfather talked about being in "camp." My grandmother told a story of working at the hospital in "camp" and helping to deliver twins. She was always beaming with pride when she recalled the event. My grandfather told fun and playful stories of playing baseball with friends and stories of pride and accomplishment when talking and negotiating with the MPs [military police] in "camp." It sounded wonderful to my naive ears. When I was in high school, I learned more about "camp," but not in my history books. In a library search, I came across a book on Japanese American internment. I was surprised and saddened, confused and curious. Why did my grandparents talk about, what seemed to be, fond memories while incarcerated? I asked my mother, and she shared that they never talked about it; she didn't ask and they didn't talk. During college, I decided to write a paper about World War II and the Japanese American internment. This was my opening, this was the permission that my grandmother and I needed to talk about "camp." We both knew she would not miss an opportunity to help me with my studies. We sat down. I asked questions, questions that hadn't been asked in a generation. She spoke in a soft, even tone, no emotion. She shared stories that had been silent, untold, invisible, buried for a generation. The stories were factual, recollections of events. I wrote down every word. She told me that law enforcement came by her house and ordered their family to prepare to leave their home, and informed them they were to pack what they were able to carry. She told me that men came into their home and sealed their drawers with beeswax. As I grew older, and more importantly as my grandmother grew older, our conversations about "camp" changed. Her voice changed, and my voice was changing. I recall asking in a defiant and troubled tone why she didn't do anything, why didn't she push back and refuse to comply, why didn't she fight back. She was quiet for several moments, and then she solemnly said, "What were we supposed to do?" Silence for several moments and then, "We had no choice." Those were painful words, I can hear them clearly, they will stay with me forever.*

*(Author)*

Intergenerational communication in Asian American families has been researched, and there is literature to support intergenerational conflicts, struggles with communication, cultural conflicts, lack of connection and understanding between generations (e.g., Nagata, 1990, 1991, 1993). For instance, "Asian-origin parents, both Japanese and Chinese, may be least likely to report conversations about discrimination or equality among groups" (Hughes et al., 2006, p. 758), and adult children of Japanese internees reported that their parents rarely, if ever, discussed the internment experience with them (e.g., Nagata, 1990, 1991, 1993; Nagata & Cheng, 2003). Young et al. (2021) found that, "familial racial socialization in Asian American families was bidirectional. Racial socialization is typically studied in the context of top-down messages from parent to child, but we found that young adults were often educating their parents about racial topics" (p. 1036). With each family and in each generation there is healing, thus, communication within and between generations may vary, but it has the potential to grow and evolve.

Some third and fourth Asian American generations may feel a sense of responsibility and a commitment to honoring their grandparents and great-grandparents by speaking the words they were not able or permitted to speak. Third- and fourth-generations have privileges and power that were not afforded to earlier generations. Groups such as Densho are "preserving Japanese American stories of the past for the generations of tomorrow" (Densho, n.d.). The Yonsei Memory Project (YMP), developed by Nikiko Masumoto, Brynn Saito, and Patricia Miye Wakida (2017), was created "to generate dialogue connecting the WWII incarceration of the Japanese American community with civil liberties struggles" (Yonsei Memory Project, n.d.). These organizations open up dialogue between generations, and with future generations, to ensure the stories of Asian Americans are remembered, retold, and persevered.

## Searching for Identity

> Chris Iijima said, "Asian American identity was only constructed as a means to organize other Asians for political purposes, to highlight aspects of racism, to escape the hegemony of Whites in progressive movements, to support other progressive racial formations, to establish alternative forms of looking at society/history ... I'm hoping that someday racial identity becomes a political identity again–not an ethnic marker.
>
> (Maeda, 2009, p. 141)

Current and future generations of Asian Americans have the opportunity to learn from their ancestors and from their own experiences as well as from researchers on Asian American ethnic identity. Constructions of Asian American identity are found within the self and consider the relationship of Asian Americans with the dominant culture. Issues of culture, context, politics, and history must be considered as Asian Americans struggle to "find their place." They "must educate themselves and initiate racial meaning-making in their families" (Young et al., 2021, p. 1027) and acknowledge the tension and confusion related to where one "fits" in the dominant culture, in one's own culture, and the social justice and activist-oriented movements. Approaching Asian American ethnic identity as a sociocultural and political process provides openings and space for the evolving dialogue and experience of Asian American identity in third and fourth generations.

## Personal Connection to the Topic

I am a Yonsei fourth-generation Japanese American, and I am biracial. My mother is Sansei, a third-generation Japanese American, and my dad is white. My parents divorced when I was eight years old, and I was raised primarily by my mother with the influence and support of her parents and cousins. In the early 1980s, my mom moved us to a new school in a new city. I can still remember walking into the school and seeing the faces of the other students and their parents. They looked the same: two white parents with white children. There were very few families who looked like mine. I think back and picture my family … absent father, a mother who looked different (Japanese American/Asian), and four children who didn't look like the mother. I was not quite sure who I was or who I was supposed to become.

I have always considered myself close to my maternal grandmother. She represented stability and constancy, an adult figure who did not expect anything of me, but was always there. She was predictable and safe, I always knew what to expect from her…good meals, sweet treats, late nights, and a comfort and acceptance that is not promised in most relationships. Grandma Heide ("*He-De*") was not a woman of many words, but her strength and sense of charity were evident. One would not go to her home without leaving with something, and she never visited someone without leaving them with a meal or special treat.

My grandmother did not talk about the internment (aka "camp") unless someone asked. During college, I remember writing a report on the Japanese American internment, and she was ready to assist by sharing stories from "camp." She spoke in a matter of fact way about how her family was given little time to pack their belongings, taking only what they could carry. She shared stories of working in the camp hospital, which block she lived in, and what she did when she left "camp." As we grew older, our relationship and her stories about "camp" changed. I will never forget one Thanksgiving while I was in graduate school and talking with my grandparents about camp. My grandfather was talking about playing baseball in camp, and I asked a question I had never dared to ask before: "Was everything really that great, was everything that fun?" The question landed like a ton of bricks, and I immediately felt it. There was silence for what felt like several minutes, then my grandmother spoke: "No." No? No.

Even though I knew the answer, I asked, "Why didn't you do anything about it." I knew we were in an unfamiliar place in our relationship. Up until this moment, I only listened and asked reflective questions about "camp." This was different, I was different, and I knew she was different. She was getting older and there was some sort of space between us that gave me permission to ask different questions. I knew that if I did not ask, the experiences and stories would be lost. She answered: "What were we supposed to do? We had no choice but to make the best of it." Her words pierced my soul and broke my heart, they also gave me a glimpse into her strength and courage and provided me with a deeper understanding of our family, her legacy, and my identity.

My racial and ethnic identity has always been fluid, and it has shifted over the last 47 years. There have been times when I have identified as Japanese American, times when I have identified as biracial, times when I have identified as a person of color, and times when I was silent in my racial and ethnic identity. There have been many times when others have identified my race and ethnicity.

## Clinical Case Example

Identity is complicated and complex, and it changes and responds to self, context, and others. Issues related to racial identity are important to consider when working with clients as racial and ethnic identity processes may provide insights into a socioculturally attuned understanding of client concerns and problems and provide the therapist with useful direction for clinical interventions. The following case of Mary and her family provides an overview of how a couple, marital, and family therapist might approach their work with a clinical case. It is important to note that despite one's theoretical orientation, issues of (1) racial identity, (2) family migration legacies, (3) racism and justice, (4) race-related trauma and resilience, and (5) intergenerational communication and connections may be integrated into any clinicians' assessment and intervention.

Kazue is a third-generation Japanese American married woman in her 40s, and she is concerned about her 13-year-old daughter, Mary. Mary started junior high school several months ago, and her attendance at school has been inconsistent. Mary is described as shy, withdrawn, anxious, and depressed, and her grades have recently dropped. Mary reports having few friends, not "fitting in," and she reverted to sleeping with her mother two months ago.

Kazue is married to Thomas, a white male in his early 50s; they met in high school and they have been married for 15 years. They struggled with infertility issues for several years; however, after two miscarriages, they had Mary. Mary is their only child. Kazue has two siblings, an older brother and an older sister. Her parents are married and they reside in a neighboring town. Kazue's parents are retired and were caring for her grandmother until her grandmother's death last year. Her grandfather died three years ago. Thomas' parents divorced when he was in middle school, and he lived between both houses as an adolescent.

He has no siblings. Thomas' father remarried and his mother remained single. Thomas' grandparents died several years ago. Thomas describes a distant relationship with his family and stated that they rarely visit.

Kazue contacted a local community-based agency for counseling services for Mary as the family has been dealing with grief and loss, developmental changes, aging parents, and upcoming retirement, and more recently, Mary's anxiety, depression, and struggles at school.

### Treatment Process

The therapist at the community-based agency is a Filipino American married male and parent to two young children. He meets with the mother, Kazue, and daughter, Mary, and observes Mary's shy and quiet demeanor. Kazue and Mary sit close to each other, and Kazue speaks throughout most of the session sharing her concerns about Mary. Mary listens, keeps her head and eyes down, and occasionally and briefly glances up when someone is speaking. The therapist invites Thomas to join the next session, But Kazue does not believe he will be able to attend due to a busy work schedule.

During the next session, Kazue and Mary are present and Kazue reports that Thomas is unable to attend due to his "busy work schedule." The therapist greets the family and inquires about the week, and Mary is quiet while Kazue reports many of the same concerns reported in the first session. The therapist inquires more about school as this was a focus of Kazue's concerns, and Mary continues to appear disengaged. Mary shrugs her shoulders when questions are posed, and the therapist decides to construct a family genogram. The genogram uncovers much information about family members in multiple generations and the therapist inquires about race and ethnicity.

### Racial Identities

The family's racial and ethnic identity includes maternal Japanese American ancestry and Thomas' white, European background. Mary is biracial, Japanese American and white, and she is fourth-generation, Yonsei, and Kazue is Sansei. Kazue's mother and father, Nisei generation, are retired, and Kazue states that she is close to her parents. Her parents were caring for her grandmother who died last year. Kazue reports that Thomas is not close to his family and he denies a racial history.

### Family Migration Legacies

The therapist learns that Kazue's grandparents migrated to the United States in the late 1800s. Her grandfather worked as a farm laborer, and her grandmother immigrated with her family to the United States. Her grandparents met and married in the early 1940s. After a few short years of marriage, the family was forced to relocate to Poston, Arizona, where they were incarcerated in Poston Internment Camp for three years.

The therapist spends time during the next several sessions making reference to the genogram and further exploring family history, family migration stories, and how the family engages with and negotiates issues of race and ethnicity. Kazue is noticeably uncomfortable with the topic and she often provides short responses. On a few occasions, she is quiet and then attempts to deflect the therapist's questions and shift the conversation. Interestingly, Mary seems more engaged in the questioning and looks up at her mother, awaiting her mother's response.

The genogram and the therapist's attention to issues of race and family legacies uncover rarely discussed issues of racism, grief and loss, and family communication barriers. As the sessions progress, mother and daughter seem more engaged and comfortable in the therapy sessions.

Kazue calls the agency before the next scheduled session and shares that there was an incident at Mary's school. She states that school officials reported an anti-Asian hate incident at the school, but she provides few details. Kazue expresses concern about Mary, and the therapist agrees to address the incident at the next session.

During the next session, Kazue reports that Mary missed many days of school since the "incident at school." The therapist listens to the concerns and notices Mary is tearful. Mary and Kazue share little about the incident, and both seem uncomfortable with the conversation. The therapist goes back to the genogram and inquires about the family's experience with racism and oppression.

### Racism and Justice

Kazue initially denies experiences of racism; however, the therapist uses the genogram to explore family history of racism related to the Japanese American internment during World War II. Kazue shares "the little" she knows about when her grandparents were incarcerated and their time in "camp." As Kazue recalls her grandparent's stories, Mary listens intently to the words. "My grandmother had my Auntie while they were in camp. After the war, they returned to their hometown, but they didn't stay. I think they must have been ashamed. Their community continued with life during the years they were gone. It was too hard for them to stay, so they left." Kazue shared what "little" she knew, but there was much about the incarceration that was never discussed. The therapist, however, was able to name and reflect on instances of racism and injustice that continued after the war.

The exploration of the family's history of racism and oppression inspired conversation on the current "incident at the school," the anti-Asian hate incident at Mary's school. Kazue reported that a group of kids vandalized the school lunchroom with racist, anti-Asian words. As Kazue spoke, Mary was quiet and looked down, and she became tearful when Kazue turned to her to confirm the story. Mary was unresponsive and tearful, and Kazue continued with other similar incidents that occurred at the school over the last few months. The therapist connected the grandparent's fear, shame, and humiliation with Mary's situation at school. This was a shift in the therapy and led to discussion on racism and intergenerational communication.

### Intergenerational Communication

Discussion of intergenerational communication as it related to current and historical issues of racism increased the emotional intensity in sessions, though Mary and Kazue continued to remain engaged in therapy sessions. The conversations uncovered grief and loss after the death of Mary's great-grandmother and Kazue's grandmother. Grief and loss associated with the incarceration of their family during World War II was also acknowledged. Conversations on intergenerational communication also uncovered Kazue and Mary's close and connected relationship, despite the difficulty over the last few months. The therapist also learned that Kazue is emotionally close to her mother and she was close to her grandmother. Interestingly, Thomas has little to no communication with his family of origin, besides biannual phone calls with some members of his family.

### Search for Identity

At this point in therapy and due to scheduling conflicts, the therapist meets with Mary for several sessions without her mother. During these sessions, Mary opens up about her relationship with her grandmother. She shares that she learned much about her "Japanese side" during the last several sessions, and she has been thinking about how unfair her grandmother was treated. She shares that she is concerned about the recent events at her school, and she is worried about how others see her. She expresses a sense of shame and also a sense of pride in her racial identity. She expresses confusion over her racial identity and she does not understand that some people do not know She is Japanese.

The therapist shares these concerns with Kazue and they discuss ways to support Mary's racial identity development. The therapist makes several suggestions, including exploring family history through internment camp monuments and other public resources (e.g., https://www.archives.gov/education/lessons/japanese-relocation; https://www.postonpreservation.org/; https://www.nps.gov/tule/index.htm), bibliotherapy (e.g., Loh-Hagan's *What is the Model Minority Myth?*, 2022), and connecting with organizations that are committed to preserving Japanese American history of incarceration (e.g., https://densho.org/). In addition, the therapist posed several different questions to Mary and allowed her to respond to the questions that seemed most "important": *How do you understand and talk about your racial identity? How do you want to identify yourself racially? What gets in the way? Are there times when your racial identity means more and times when it does not matter? Are there times when your race is identified and defined by others? What do you think about those times? How do incidents like the one at your school impact your view and experience of your identity? How does your grandmother and family migration stories impact your racial identity?* The rich conversations about Mary's racial identity and her understanding of and relationship with family migration stories and experiences of racism shifted the therapeutic relationship.

As therapy continued with this family and in addition to the identity and racial issues addressed above, the therapist discussed several topics during the course of therapy, including how the parenting relationship is informed by Asian American identity, values, and intergenerational strengths and traumas (e.g., Tuttle et al., 2012). It is important to note that this case discussion does not adequately attend to issues of parenting, safety and risk, inclusion and integration of both parents in the treatment process and Thomas' lack of involvement (e.g., treatment configuration; who to work with and when), assessment and treatment planning, self-of-therapist, specific couple and family therapy theories, and other relevant treatment considerations. Therapists must consider these issues and relevant legal and ethical considerations when applying these ideas.

Therapists working with Asian American identified individuals, such as Mary and her family, are able to consider how racial and ethnic identities intersect with presenting problems, such as depression, anxiety, grief, and loss. Racial identity, family migration legacies, racism and justice, race-related trauma and resilience, and intergenerational communication and connections may be salient topics to include in clinical assessment and intervention. In this case, Kazue is concerned about Mary; however, in the treatment process, the presenting concerns are reduced through an exploration of Mary's Asian American identity struggles, Kazue's response to grief by distancing from grandparent's migration stories, and Thomas' lack of connection with Mary's biracial identity process. Genograms may be helpful in tracing racial histories and examining migration stories and race-related trauma, and intergenerational patterns of resilience and empowerment may be used as sources of support and connection between and within generations. These therapeutic considerations may expose and support the complex, evolving ethnic identity process for Asian Americans.

## Reflection Questions

### Questions for the Therapist

- How does your ethnic and racial socialization impact your personal and professional relationships? How does it impact your clinical work? What values do you integrate into your clinical work? What issues of race-related trauma impact your clinical work?

- How do historical sociopolitical issues impact your personal and professional relationships? How do they impact your identity?
- How do you manage intergenerational race-related trauma? How does it show up in your personal and professional relationships?
- How has your racial and ethnic identity shifted and changed? How do you experience these changes, if any?
- How does your power and privilege intersect with Asian Americans' identity? How might you interrupt potentially damaging effects of your power and privilege?

### Questions for Therapy

- How do you understand and talk about your racial identity? How do you want to identify yourself racially? What gets in the way?
- Are there times when your racial identity means more and times when it does not matter? Are there times when your race is identified and defined by others? How do you experience this?
- How do anti-Asian hate incidents impact you and others around you?
- How do your family migration stories impact your racial identity?

## References

Asian Society. (2023, June 5). *Asian Americans then and now*. https://asiasociety.org/education/asian-americans-then-and-now

Attias-Donfut, C. (2015). Hansen's law. In J. Stone, R.M. Dennis, & P. Rizova (Eds.), *The Wiley Blackwell encyclopedia of race, ethnicity and nationalism*. Wiley. https://doi.org/10.1002/9781118663202.wberen478

Attias-Donfut, C. (2016). Older migrants' ageing and dying: An intergenerational perspective. In U. Karl & S. Torres (Eds.), *Ageing in contexts of migration* (pp. 83–95). Routledge.

Densho. (2023, June 5). *Preserving Japanese American stories of the past for generations of tomorrow*. https://densho.org/

Goon, C., Bruce, T. A., Lun, J., Lai, G. Y., Chu, S., & Le, P. (2022). Examining Asian American leadership gap and inclusion issues with federal employee data: Recommendations for inclusive workforce analytic practices. *Frontiers in Research Metrics and Analysis, 7*, 1–14. https://doi.org/10.3389/frma.2022.958750

Han, S., Riddel, J. R., & Piquero, A. R. (2023). Anti-Asian American hate crimes spike during the early stages of the COVID-19 pandemic. *Journal of Interpersonal Violence, 38*(3–4), 3513–3533. https://doi.org/10.1177/08862605221107056

Hughes, D., Rodriguez, J., Smith, E. P., Johnson, D. J., Stevenson, H. C., & Spicer, P. (2006). Parents' ethnic–racial socialization practices: A review of research and

directions for future study. *Developmental Psychology, 42*(5), 747–770. https://doi
.org/10.1037/0012-1649.42.5.747

Kim, J. (1981). Processes of Asian American identity development: A study of Japanese
American women's perceptions of their struggle to achieve positive identities as
Americans of Asian 7 ancestry. [Doctoral Dissertation University of Massachusetts
Amherst]. Available from Proquest. AAI8118010.

Kim, J. (2001). Asian American racial identity theory. In C. L. Wijeyesinghe & B. W.
Jackson III (Eds.), *New perspectives on racial identity development: A theoretical and
practical anthology* (pp. 138–161). New York University Press

Kwan, K.-L. K., & Sodowsky, G. R. (1997). Internal and external ethnic identity and
their correlates: A study of Chinese American immigrants. *Journal of Multicultural
Counseling and Development,* 25(1), 51–67. https://doi.org/10.1002/j.2161-1912
.1997.tb00315.x

Lee, J., & Sheng, D. (2023). The Asian American assimilation paradox. *Journal or
Ethnic and Migration Studies, 50*(1), 68–94. https://doi.org/10.1080/1369183X.2023
.2183965.

Lee, J. F. J. (1992). *Asian Americans: Oral histories of first to fourth generation
Americans from China, the Philippines, Japan, India, the Pacific Islands, Vietnam
and Cambodia.* The New Press.

Lee, S., & Rose, R. (2022). Unexpected benefits: New resilience among intergenerational
Asian-Americans during the COVID-19 pandemic. *Social Work with Groups, 45*(1),
61–67. https://doi.org/10.1080/01609513.2020.1868705

Loh-Hagan, V. (2022). *What is the model minority myth?* Cherry Lake Publishing Group.

Lui, M., Geron, K., & Lai, T. (2008). *The snake dance of Asian American activism.*
Lexington Books.

Maeda, D. J. (2009). *Chains of Babylon: The rise of Asian America.* University of
Minnesota Press.

Maeda, D. J. (2012). *Rethinking the Asian American movement.* Routledge.

Masumoto, N., Saito, B. & Miye Wakida, P. (2017). *Yonsei memory project.* https://www
.yonseimemoryproject.com/

Nagata, D. K. (1990). The Japanese-American internment: Perceptions of moral
community, fairness, and redress. *Journal of Social Issues, 46*(1), 133–146. https://
doi.org/10.1111/j.1540-4560.1990.tb00277.x

Nagata, D. K. (1991). Transgenerational impact of the Japanese American internment:
Clinical issues in working with children of former internees. *Psychotherapy, 28,* 121–
128. https://doi.org/10.1037/0033-3204.28.1.121

Nagata, D. K. (1993). *Legacy of injustice: Exploring the cross-generational impact of the
Japanese American internment.* Plenum Press.

Nagata, D. K., & Cheng, W. J. Y. (2003). Intergenerational communication of race-related
trauma by Japanese American former internees. *American Journal of Orthopsychiatry,
73*(3), 266–278. https://doi.org/10.1037/0002-9432.73.3.266

Newton, B. J., Buck, E. B., Kunimura, D. T., Colfer, C. P., & Scholsberg, D. (1988).
Ethnic identity among Japanese-Americans in Hawaii: A critique of Hansen's third-
generation return hypothesis. *International Journal of Intercultural Relations, 12*(4),
305–315. https://doi.org/10.1016/0147-1767(88)90028-4Get rights and content

Pew Research. (2021). https://www.pewresearch.org/short-reads/2021/04/29/key-facts -about-asian-americans/

Stop AAPI Hate (2023, June 5). *Our mission.* https://stopaapihate.org/about/

Sue, D. W., & Sue, D. (1990). *Counseling the culturally different: Theory and practice* (2nd ed.). John Wiley & Sons.

Tuttle, A., Knudson-Martin, C., & Kim. L. (2012). Parenting as relationship: A framework for assessment and practice. *Family Process, 51*, 73–89. https://doi.org/10.1111/j .1545-5300.2012.01383.x.

Wallace, N. (2017, May 8). *Yellow power: The origins of Asian American.* https://densho .org/catalyst/asian-american-movement/

Wei, W. (1993). *The Asian American movement.* Temple University Press.

Yonsei Memory Project. (2023, June 5). *Awakening the archives of Japanese American history through arts and story-telling, memory-mapping, and intergenerational dialogue.* https://www.yonseimemoryproject.com/

Yoo, H. C., Gabriel, A. K., Atkin, A. L., Matriano, R. & Akhter. S. (2021). A new measure of Asian American racial identity ideological values (AARIIV): Unity solidarity, and transnational critical consciousness. *Asian American Journal of Psychology*, 12(4), 317–332. https://doi.org/10.1037/aap0000256

Young, J. L., Kim, H., & Golojuch, L. (2021). Race was something we didn't talk about: Racial socialization in Asian American families. *Family Relations, 70*, 1027–1039. https://doi.org/10.1111/fare.12495

# Acknowledgments

It is a gift that the two of us met as doctoral students and had the opportunity to share our educational heritage through the faculty we trained under at Loma Linda University. Our vision for this book would not have been possible without Carmen Knudson-Martin's stalwart mentorship throughout our careers. From close involvement in her Socio-Emotional Relationship Therapy research group to the many years we have shared writing, presenting, and serving in the field together, we thank you for investing in us and for your humility in welcoming, inviting, integrating, and centering the voices of your students of color. We are also grateful to our beloved LLU colleagues whose collaboration and friendship have empowered and sustained us in our development as Asian American women faculty (Justine D'Arrigo, Lisa Esmiol Wilson, Lindsey Nice).

Throughout the writing and editing of this book, we have held close our relationships with Asian American colleagues, mentors, and students/supervisees. Even if they were brief touchpoints at a conference or having you as one of the only Asian American students in a class, your voice and experiences have shaped this book.

We want to acknowledge our publisher Routledge for seeing the timely need of giving voice to Asian American authors and clinicians. Thank you for creating this space for visibility.

In our families' complex migration journeys – forced and chosen displacements – we are grateful for the lives we could build on the land of our Indigenous siblings. Our own post-migration stories and the writing of this book have taken place on the land of the Gabrieleno (Tongva) peoples, Serrano (Maara'yam) peoples, Chemehuevi (Nuwu) peoples, Yuhaaviatam (San Manuel nation), Multnomah, Kathlamet, Clackamas, Tumwater, and Watalala bands of the Chinook, the Tualatin Kalapuya, and many other Indigenous nations of the N'chi-Wana (Columbia) River.

For me (Lana) this book holds as much personal meaning as it does professional, and there are many people, whether they know it or not, who have played direct and indirect roles to actualize it. To some of my dearest MFT friends and colleagues from the early days: Marlene Ferreras, Kirstee Williams, Lisa Esmiol-Wilson, Laura Montane, Martha Laughlin, Kate Warner, and Jennifer Lambert-Shute. Each of you served a pivotal role in my development and identity as an Asian American MFT, and I thank you for your friendship and collegiality. Rafe McCullough, Lina Darwich, and Elena Diamond, my generational colleagues, thank you for reality checking and providing grounding and safety in academic space. The countless conversations about all things – life, relationships, identities, and our work in the academe, sustain me. Your musings, reflections, and passions have inspired and fueled me to also pursue mine. To Barbara Hernandez, thank you for your unwavering belief in me, your mentorship throughout the years, and for modeling what it looks like to lead with a strong back and soft heart.

To my husband, Aidan Wright, thank you for sharing the reins and tag teaming every day to ensure that our world keeps spinning. My children, Isla and Lael, you bring so much meaning and laughter to umma's life. It is my greatest privilege to be your mama and watch you become your own people. As I reflected on halmi and halbi's immigrant experience while writing and editing this book, I also dreamed of your lives today and a version of the world that I hope books like this can help create for tomorrow.

To my parents, Kim Dae Hi and Kim Hyun Soon, no words can express my deep appreciation for your endless sacrifice, unconditional support, and steadfast love. I admire the strength you had to migrate to a country without much, knowing little about the language and culture, while holding hope for a better future. You have both taught me so much about courage, tenacity, hard work, generosity, humility, and faith. I am forever grateful for the life I get to live because of you. I hope this book pays homage to the lives you live.

To my brothers, Michael and Kevin Kim, thanks for all your love, support, and understanding. You know and experience a version of our family's post-migration legacy that only you could get as second-generation siblings, and it means so much that we get to raise our third-generation children together. In addition, endless thanks to my cousin siblings, the Cha sisters and Karen unni, for helping to foster and maintain extended family connection today into the future. Bong Sun halmoni's spirit and legacy are felt whenever all of us gather together and I am grateful to you as cousin siblings for providing continuity of kinship and cultural identity. Thank you also to all the Kim eemos for hosting the many family get-togethers throughout the years, where halmoni's masterful Korean cooking skills were passed down and her generous spirit and love for others was instilled.

I also thank and acknowledge my Foremost grandparents, Muriel and Eddie Luca and their children and grandchildren, for creating the unimaginable opportunity for my dad to come to Canada in 1970, with no conditions attached. I regard that as one of the purest forms of brotherly love, racial allyship, and social justice in action. Thank you for accepting my dad and our family into your family. We will forever be grateful.

And to my co-author and editor, Jessica, thank you for the privilege to dream and launch this book with you. The personal and professional conversations we have shared while envisioning this book and long before it have been some of the most grounding and meaningful ones in my career. May the themes carried in this book inspire healing conversations throughout our communities.

When I (Jessica) think about what in my life has given birth to this book, it is undoubtedly the impact of queer friends and women of color. The developing of my own critical consciousness was catalyzed in the season of being an AAMFT minority fellow; thank you Mudita Rastogi for being the first and only Asian American mentor I've ever had and for your wise counsel to marry a feminist partner. DeAnna, Yajaira, and Christiana: your strong voices as WOC inspired me to find my own. Dana, our friendship has been a beautiful safe place since the start of my academic career to unpack all the things. Jeney PH, Sandy K, Julie T, and Janna L: each of you are Asian American women who have modeled your own ways of using your voice to speak for our and other marginalized communities – an inspiration to me finding my own way. Justine: our friendship and who you are has been one of the greatest gifts of my life.

Barbara Hernandez: from the beginning until now, your encouragement and support has shaped the trajectory of my scholarship in every way. Your believing in and seeing me is a tremendous gift. Amy, Zane, and Saúl: who each of you are and our friendships have brought so much repair and healing to my life. Cedric: your respect and support has meant so much to me and has fueled me through the writing of this book. Fuller AAC: until now, I had never known the gift of having our own racial/ethnic center as part of my faculty academic experience; it has been life-changing to feel like I belong, am known, and that together we have something important to offer – each of you has contributed to the courage I needed to write the words in this book.

SHHS Azn FloWeRs: we have been sisters and mothers to one another across a lifetime. What a gift to journey through our second-gen adolescence and young adulthood together, and to now be able to together make sense of our first-gen parents and raise our third-gen children. I carry our stories and our secure base of connection into all that I do. Recalibrated Performance coaches and friends: your encouragement and inspiration to pursue the strongest version of myself over this last year has transformed who I am and know I can be.

To Chen and Jan *ahmas*: in our families' post-migration stories, you are the matriarchs from whom we have inherited the capacity to *jím-nāi*. Thank you for raising our families with such abundant love, grace, and fortitude.

Mom and Dad: Jackie and I are so blessed to have the most amazing parents. Our capacity to be our best, have dreams and hopes, and feel secure in ourselves is because of the lifetime of unconditional love, relentless support, and modeled sacrifice you have given us. Who we are is because you have instilled integrity, perseverance, respect, and courage in us. Mei: it is such a precious gift to go through this life together; I love that we get to bear our family's legacy together, raise our children together, and encourage and inspire each other in our dreams as Taiwanese American sisters.

Andre: the one I get to run this race with. Thank you for always supporting my career and amplifying my voice. I admire your commitment to give your all for the sake of intergenerational healing and liberation. Thank you for loving us through your courageous pursuit of all that is good, right, and just.

Justus and Liberty: it is absolute pure joy to be your mama and I love the fire in each of you. J, your tenacity, heart of justice, and compassion inspire me. L, your spunk, resoluteness, and unapologetic existence is light and fresh air. You are both already living out what I have dreamed for you.

Lana, my co-editor/author, but most significantly, my friend. There is no way this book would have happened without you. One of the greatest gifts of my career is our friendship; to carry together the painful invisibility of being Asian American women in academia but then to see and know one another so profoundly in being working moms of young children, and all the while doing it all with such grace and competence. Through this experience, I feel all the more connected to your ancestors and mine, and I imagine that they would be proud of what we are doing with our inheritance.

# Index